S0-BJR-165

Trauma, Stress, and Resilience Among Sexual Minority Women: Rising Like the Phoenix

Trauma, Stress, and Resilience Among Sexual Minority Women: Rising Like the Phoenix has been co-published simultaneously as *Journal of Lesbian Studies*, Volume 7, Number 4 2003.

The *Journal of Lesbian Studies* Monographic "Separates"

Below is a list of "separates," which in serials librarianship means a special issue simultaneously published as a special journal issue or double-issue *and* as a "separate" hardbound monograph. (This is a format which we also call a "DocuSerial.")

"Separates" are published because specialized libraries or professionals may wish to purchase a specific thematic issue by itself in a format which can be separately cataloged and shelved, as opposed to purchasing the journal on an on-going basis. Faculty members may also more easily consider a "separate" for classroom adoption.

"Separates" are carefully classified separately with the major book jobbers so that the journal tie-in can be noted on new book order slips to avoid duplicate purchasing.

You may wish to visit Haworth's website at . . .

http://www.HaworthPress.com

. . . to search our online catalog for complete tables of contents of these separates and related publications.

You may also call 1-800-HAWORTH (outside US/Canada: 607-722-5857), or Fax 1-800-895-0582 (outside US/Canada: 607-771-0012), or e-mail at:

docdelivery@haworthpress.com

Trauma, Stress, and Resilence Among Sexual Minority Women: Rising Like the Phoenix, edited by Kimberly F. Balsam, PhD (Vol. 7, No. 4, 2003). *Provides a first-hand look at the victimization experiences that lesbian and bisexual women face as well as how they work through these challenges and emerge resilient.*

Latina Lesbian Writers and Artists, edited by María Dolores Costa, PhD (Vol. 7, No. 3, 2003). *"A fascinating journey through the Latina lesbian experience. It brings us stories of exile, assimilation, and conflict of cultures. The book takes us to the Midwest, New York, Chicana Borderlands, Mexico, Argentina, and Spain. It succeeds at showing the diversity within the Latina lesbian experience through deeply feminist testimonials of life and struggle." (Susana Cook, performance artist and playwright)*

Lesbian Rites: Symbolic Acts and the Power of Community, edited by Ramona Faith Oswald, PhD (Vol. 7, No. 2, 2003). *"Informative, enlightening, and well written . . . illuminates the range of lesbian ritual behavior in a creative and thorough manner. Ramona Faith Oswald and the contributors to this book have done scholars and students of ritual studies an important service by demonstrating the power, pervasiveness, and performative nature of lesbian ritual practices." (Cele Otnes, PhD, Associate Professor, Department of Business Administration, University of Illinois)*

Mental Health Issues for Sexual Minority Women: Re-Defining Women's Mental Health, edited by Tonda L. Hughes, RN, PhD, FAAN, Carrol Smith, RN, MS and Alice Dan, PhD (Vol. 7, No. 1, 2003). *A rare look at mental health issues for lesbians and other sexual minority women.*

Addressing Homophobia and Heterosexism on College Campuses, edited by Elizabeth P. Cramer, PhD (Vol. 6, No. 3/4, 2002). *A practical guide to creating LGBT-supportive environments on college campuses.*

Femme/Butch: New Considerations of the Way We Want to Go, edited by Michelle Gibson and Deborah T. Meem (Vol. 6, No. 2, 2002). *"Disrupts the fictions of heterosexual norms. . . . A much-needed examiniation of the ways that butch/femme identitites subvert both heteronormativity and 'expected' lesbian behavior." (Patti Capel Swartz, PhD, Assistant Professor of English, Kent State University)*

Lesbian Love and Relationships, edited by Suzanna M. Rose, PhD (Vol. 6, No. 1, 2002). *"Suzanna Rose's collection of 13 essays is well suited to prompting serious contemplation and discussion about lesbian lives and how they are–or are not–different from others. . . . Interesting and useful for debunking some myths, confirming others, and reaching out into new territories that were previously unexplored." (Lisa Keen, BA, MFA, Senior Political Correspondent, Washington Blade)*

Everyday Mutinies: Funding Lesbian Activism, edited by Nanette K. Gartrell, MD, and Esther D. Rothblum, PhD (Vol. 5, No. 3, 2001). *"Any lesbian who fears she'll never find the money, time, or support for her work can take heart from the resourcefulness and dogged determination of the contributors to this book. Not only do these inspiring stories provide practical tips on making dreams come true, they offer an informal history of lesbian political activism since World War II." (Jane Futcher, MA, Reporter,* Marin Independent Journal, *and author of* Crush, Dream Lover, *and* Promise Not to Tell)

Lesbian Studies in Aotearoa/New Zealand, edited by Alison J. Laurie (Vol. 5, No. 1/2, 2001). *These fascinating studies analyze topics ranging from the gender transgressions of women passing as men in order to work and marry as they wished to the effects of coming out on modern women's health.*

Lesbian Self-Writing: The Embodiment of Experience, edited by Lynda Hall (Vol. 4, No. 4, 2000). *"Probes the intersection of love for words and love for women. . . . Luminous, erotic, evocative." (Beverly Burch, PhD, psychotherapist and author,* Other Women: Lesbian/Bisexual Experience and Psychoanalytic Views of Women *and* On Intimate Terms: The Psychology of Difference in Lesbian Relationships)

'Romancing the Margins'? Lesbian Writing in the 1990s, edited by Gabriele Griffin, PhD (Vol. 4, No. 2, 2000). *Explores lesbian issues through the mediums of books, movies, and poetry and offers readers critical essays that examine current lesbian writing and discuss how recent movements have tried to remove racist and anti-gay themes from literature and movies.*

From Nowhere to Everywhere: Lesbian Geographies, edited by Gill Valentine, PhD (Vol. 4, No. 1, 2000). *"A significant and worthy contribution to the ever growing literature on sexuality and space. . . . A politically significant volume representing the first major collection on lesbian geographies. . . . I will make extensive use of this book in my courses on social and cultural geography and sexuality and space." (Jon Binnie, PhD, Lecturer in Human Geography, Liverpool, John Moores University, United Kingdom)*

Lesbians, Levis and Lipstick: The Meaning of Beauty in Our Lives, edited by Jeanine C. Cogan, PhD, and Joanie M. Erickson (Vol. 3, No. 4, 1999). *Explores lesbian beauty norms and the effects these norms have on lesbian women.*

Lesbian Sex Scandals: Sexual Practices, Identities, and Politics, edited by Dawn Atkins, MA (Vol. 3, No. 3, 1999). *"Grounded in material practices, this collection explores confrontation and coincidence among identity politics, 'scandalous' sexual practices, and queer theory and feminism. . . . It expands notions of lesbian identification and lesbian community." (Maria Pramaggiore, PhD, Assistant Professor, Film Studies, North Carolina State University, Raleigh)*

The Lesbian Polyamory Reader: Open Relationships, Non-Monogamy, and Casual Sex, edited by Marcia Munson and Judith P. Stelboum, PhD (Vol. 3, No. 1/2, 1999). *"Offers reasonable, logical, and persuasive explanations for a style of life I had not seriously considered before. . . . A terrific read." (Beverly Todd, Acquisitions Librarian, Estes Park Public Library, Estes Park, Colorado)*

Living "Difference": Lesbian Perspectives on Work and Family Life, edited by Gillian A. Dunne, PhD (Vol. 2, No. 4, 1998). *"A fascinating, groundbreaking collection. . . . Students and professionals in psychiatry, psychology, sociology, and anthropology will find this work extremely useful and thought provoking." (Nanette K. Gartrell, MD, Associate Clinical Professor of Psychiatry, University of California at San Francisco Medical School)*

Acts of Passion: Sexuality, Gender, and Performance, edited by Nina Rapi, MA, and Maya Chowdhry, MA (Vol. 2, No. 2/3, 1998). *"This significant and impressive publication draws together a diversity of positions, practices, and polemics in relation to postmodern lesbian performance and puts them firmly on the contemporary cultural map." (Lois Keidan, Director of Live Arts, Institute of Contemporary Arts, London, United Kingdom)*

Gateways to Improving Lesbian Health and Health Care: Opening Doors, edited by Christy M. Ponticelli, PhD (Vol. 2, No. 1, 1997). *"An unprecedented collection that goes to the source for powerful and poignant information on the state of lesbian health care." (Jocelyn C. White, MD, Assistant Professor of Medicine, Oregon Health Sciences University; Faculty, Portland Program in General Internal Medicine, Legacy Portland Hospitals, Portland, Oregon)*

Classics in Lesbian Studies, edited by Esther Rothblum, PhD (Vol. 1, No. 1, 1996). *"Brings together a collection of powerful chapters that cross disciplines and offer a broad vision of lesbian lives across race, age, and community." (Michele J. Eliason, PhD, Associate Professor, College of Nursing, The University of Iowa)*

Trauma, Stress, and Resilience Among Sexual Minority Women: Rising Like the Phoenix

Kimberly F. Balsam, PhD
Editor

Trauma, Stress, and Resilience Among Sexual Minority Women: Rising Like the Phoenix has been co-published simultaneously as *Journal of Lesbian Studies*, Volume 7, Number 4 2003.

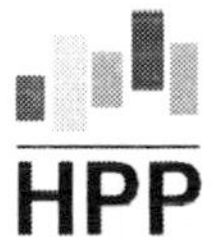

Harrington Park Press®
An Imprint of The Haworth Press, Inc.

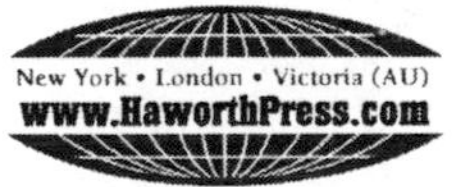

Published by

Harrington Park Press®, 10 Alice Street, Binghamton, NY 13904-1580 USA

Harrington Park Press® is an imprint of The Haworth Press, Inc., 10 Alice Street, Binghamton, NY 13904-1580 USA.

Trauma, Stress, and Resilience Among Sexual Minority Women: Rising Like the Phoenix has been co-published simultaneously as *Journal of Lesbian Studies*, Volume 7, Number 4 2003.

Cover design by Lora Wiggins

Library of Congress Cataloging-in-Publication Data

Trauma, stress, and resilience among sexual minority women : rising like the phoenix / Kimberly F. Balsam, editor.
p. cm.
"Co-published simultaneously as Journal of lesbian studies, volume 7, number 4, 2003."
Includes bibliographical references and index.
ISBN 1-56023-306-0 (hard cover : alk. paper) – ISBN 1-56023-307-9 (soft cover : alk. paper)
1. Lesbians–Psychology. 2. Bisexual women–Psychology. 3. Minority lesbians–Psychology. I. Balsam, Kimberly F. II. Journal of lesbian studies.
HQ76.25.T73 2003
306.76′63–dc22

2003018149

Indexing, Abstracting & Website/Internet Coverage

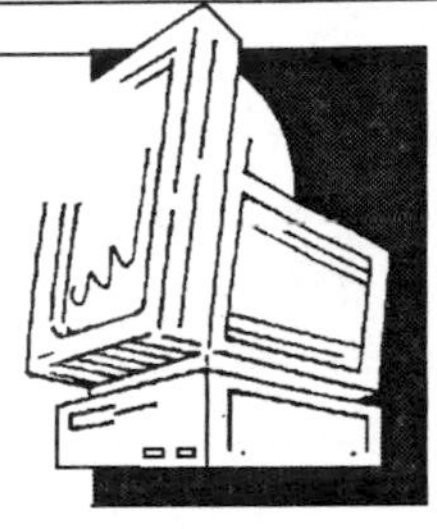

This section provides you with a list of major indexing & abstracting services. That is to say, each service began covering this periodical during the year noted in the right column. Most Websites which are listed below have indicated that they will either post, disseminate, compile, archive, cite or alter their own Website users with research-based content from this work. (This list is as current as the copyright date of this publication.)

Abstracting, Website/Indexing Coverage . . . . Year When Coverage Began

- ***Abstracts in Social Gerontology: Current Literature on Aging*** 1997
- ***CNPIEC Reference Guide: Chinese National Directory of Foreign Periodicals*** 1997
- ***Contemporary Women's Issues*** 1998
- ***e-psyche, LLC <www.e-psyche.net>*** 2001
- ***Family & Society Studies Worldwide <www.nisc.com>*** 2001
- ***Family Index Database <www.familyscholar.com>*** 2003
- ***Feminist Periodicals: A Current Listing of Contents*** 1997
- ***Gay & Lesbian Abstracts <www.nisc.com>*** 1997
- ***GenderWatch <www.slinfo.com>*** 1999
- ***HOMODOK/"Relevant" Bibliographic database, Documentation Centre for Gay & Lesbian Studies, University of Amsterdam (selective printed abstracts in "Homologie" and bibliographic computer databases covering cultural, historical, social, and political aspects of gay & lesbian topics)*** 1997
- ***IBZ International Bibliography of Periodical Literature <www.saur.de>*** 2001

(continued)

- ***IGLSS Abstracts <www.iglss.org>*** **2000**
- ***Index to Periodical Articles Related to Law*** **1997**
- ***OCLC Public Affairs Information Service <www.pais.org>*** **1997**
- ***Psychological Abstracts (PsycINFO) <www.apa.org>*** **2003**
- ***Referativnyi Zhurnal (Abstracts Journal of the All-Russian Institute of Scientific and Technical Information–in Russian)*** . . . **1997**
- ***Social Services Abstracts <www.csa.com>*** **1998**
- ***Sociological Abstracts (SA) <www.csa.com>*** **1998**
- ***Studies on Women and Gender Abstracts <www.tandf.co.uk>*** **1998**
- ***Women's Studies Index (indexed comprehensively)*** **1997**

Special Bibliographic Notes related to special journal issues (separates) and indexing/abstracting:

- indexing/abstracting services in this list will also cover material in any "separate" that is co-published simultaneously with Haworth's special thematic journal issue or DocuSerial. Indexing/abstracting usually covers material at the article/chapter level.
- monographic co-editions are intended for either non-subscribers or libraries which intend to purchase a second copy for their circulating collections.
- monographic co-editions are reported to all jobbers/wholesalers/approval plans. The source journal is listed as the "series" to assist the prevention of duplicate purchasing in the same manner utilized for books-in-series.
- to facilitate user/access services all indexing/abstracting services are encouraged to utilize the co-indexing entry note indicated at the bottom of the first page of each article/chapter/contribution.
- this is intended to assist a library user of any reference tool (whether print, electronic, online, or CD-ROM) to locate the monographic version if the library has purchased this version but not a subscription to the source journal.
- individual articles/chapters in any Haworth publication are also available through the Haworth Document Delivery Service (HDDS).

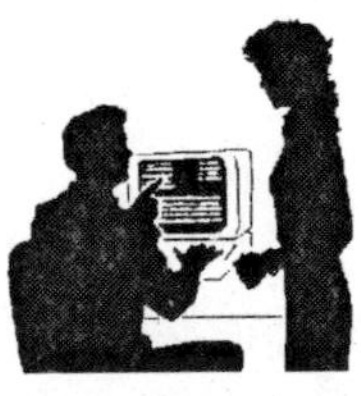

Trauma, Stress, and Resilience Among Sexual Minority Women: Rising Like the Phoenix

CONTENTS

Acknowledgments xiii

Trauma, Stress, and Resilience Among Sexual Minority Women: Rising Like the Phoenix 1
Kimberly F. Balsam

Lesbian and Bisexual Female Youths Aged 14 to 21: Developmental Challenges and Victimization Experiences 9
Anthony R. D'Augelli

Sexual Abuse in Lesbian and Bisexual Young Women: Associations with Emotional/Behavioral Difficulties, Feelings About Sexuality, and the "Coming Out" Process 31
Jennifer S. Robohm
Brian W. Litzenberger
Laurie Anne Pearlman

Abuse, Social Support, and Depression Among HIV-Positive Heterosexual, Bisexual, and Lesbian Women 49
Nina A. Cooperman
Jane M. Simoni
David W. Lockhart

Lesbian and Bisexual Women's Experiences of Victimization: Mental Health, Revictimization, and Sexual Identity Development 67
Jessica F. Morris
Kimberly F. Balsam

Triple Jeopardy and Beyond: Multiple Minority Stress and Resilience Among Black Lesbians 87
Lisa Bowleg
Jennifer Huang
Kelly Brooks
Amy Black
Gary Burkholder

Cast into the Wilderness: The Impact of Institutionalized Religion on Lesbians 109
Deana F. Morrow

Community Interventions Concerning Homophobic Violence and Partner Violence Against Lesbians 125
Suzanna M. Rose

Index 141

ABOUT THE EDITOR

Kimberly F. Balsam, PhD, is a Postdoctoral Research Fellow in the Department of Psychology at the University of Washington. She received her PhD in Clinical Psychology in 2003 from the University of Vermont. Dr. Balsam's research focuses on stress, trauma, and mental health among marginalized populations, with a special emphasis on lesbian, gay, bisexual, and transgendered (LGBT) adults. Her doctoral dissertation, "Traumatic victimization: A comparison of lesbian, gay, and bisexual adults and their heterosexual siblings," won awards from the Society for the Scientific Study of Sexuality, the Society for the Psychological Study of Social Issues, the Roy Scrivner foundation, and the Child and Adolescent Psychology Foundation. She also received a citation from the American College Personnel Association for Outstanding Contribution to Research on Lesbian, Gay, Bisexual, and Transgender Issues. Dr. Balsam has practiced psychotherapy since 1993 in a variety of settings. She has served on the Board of Directors of SafeSpace, a community organization addressing the needs of LGBT survivors of violence in Burlington, Vermont. Dr. Balsam has a special interest in promoting the career development of sexual minority graduate students in psychology and from 2000-2003 she initiated and coordinated a nationwide mentoring program for these students through the American Psychological Association-Graduate Students Committee on Lesbian, Gay, Bisexual and Transgender Concerns. Dr. Balsam lives with her partner, Kerri, in Seattle, Washington.

∞ ALL HARRINGTON PARK PRESS BOOKS
AND JOURNALS ARE PRINTED
ON CERTIFIED ACID-FREE PAPER

Acknowledgments

I wish to thank Judith Bradford, Bryan Cochran, Joanne DiPlacido, Joseph Doherty, Laura Gibson, Judith Glassgold, Debra Kaysen, Frances Kelley, Joanna Pashdag, and Dawn Szymanski for their helpful reviews of manuscripts for this volume. I would also like to extend my sincere gratitude to Esther D. Rothblum, my doctoral advisor and the editor of *Journal of Lesbian Studies,* for providing guidance in this endeavor. Finally, I want to thank my partner, Kerri Ashling, for her loving support and patience during the editing of this volume and always.

–Kimberly F. Balsam

Trauma, Stress, and Resilience Among Sexual Minority Women: Rising Like the Phoenix

Kimberly F. Balsam

In June 2002, in the midst of editing this volume, I attended a women's dance that was being held in conjunction with the annual Vermont Pride celebration. Because this was one of a few such events in this part of Northern New England, women from all over the geographical region were in attendance, and I found myself looking out into a crowd of mostly unfamiliar faces. Attending Pride events has always been a powerful emotional experience for me, as it is for many lesbian, gay, bisexual, and transgender people; yet this time I found myself reflecting on a deeper level about the implications of my academic work. Looking out at these anonymous women, I felt a sense of awe and amazement. In her own unique way, each of these women had been faced with the conflict between her own desires and those deemed "acceptable" by society. Each woman had faced, on a daily basis, the challenge of being the "other." Furthermore, given data from my dissertation (Balsam, 2002) and other recent studies (e.g., Corliss, Cochran, & Mays, 2003; Tjaden, Thoeness, & Allison, 1999), I was aware that these women, to a greater extent than their heterosexual counterparts, had also faced the trauma of interpersonal violence in their families and communities. And yet here they were, laughing, rejoicing, celebrating their pride and connection with each other. This juxtaposition struck me, and I found myself wondering about the myriad of ways that sexual

[Haworth co-indexing entry note]: "Trauma, Stress, and Resilience Among Sexual Minority Women: Rising Like the Phoenix." Balsam, Kimberly F. Co-published simultaneously in *Journal of Lesbian Studies* (Harrington Park Press, an imprint of The Haworth Press, Inc.) Vol. 7, No. 4, 2003, pp. 1-8; and: *Trauma, Stress, and Resilience Among Sexual Minority Women: Rising Like the Phoenix* (ed: Kimberly F. Balsam) Harrington Park Press, an imprint of The Haworth Press, Inc., 2003, pp. 1-8. Single or multiple copies of this article are available for a fee from The Haworth Document Delivery Service [1-800-HAWORTH, 9:00 a.m. - 5:00 p.m. (EST). E-mail address: docdelivery@haworthpress.com].

http://www.haworthpress.com/store/product.asp?sku=J155

10.1300/J155v07n04_01

minority women thrived in the face of adversity. What kinds of challenges had they faced? What did it mean for a woman already living with the stresses of homophobia to experience physical or sexual abuse? How did they make sense of their experiences? Where did their resilience come from?

Questions such as these inspired this volume. The papers brought together here provide empirical, qualitative, and theoretical perspectives on sexual minority women's experiences of trauma, stress, and resilience. The field of trauma studies has grown tremendously over the past two decades, with a strong emphasis on interpersonal victimization in the lives of women and children. In contrast, relatively little research has focused on trauma and victimization in the lives of lesbian and bisexual women. The papers in this volume further our understanding of the prevalence and impact of experiences as such as physical and sexual abuse over the lifespan. Additionally, the more ongoing, daily stresses of living as a sexual minority are explored. Recent scholarship on lesbian and bisexual women's lives has brought into focus the psychological impact of living with homophobia and heterosexism. Along these lines, the papers contained here provide valuable insights into the nature, impact, and meaning of experiences of discrimination, invisibility, and oppression. In editing this volume, I sought to explore the boundaries of our understanding of trauma by examining the intersections between trauma and oppression, between individual and cultural distress, between personal and community resilience. Accordingly, several authors examine the ways in which living with oppression might influence responses to trauma on both individual and community levels. While the context of lesbian and bisexual women's lives presents unique challenges, this context can also be fertile ground for the development of resilience. Taken together, this collection of papers highlight some important strengths found in lesbian and bisexual communities, pointing the way to future prevention and intervention strategies.

One important topic addressed in this volume concerns the prevalence of experiences of verbal, physical, and sexual abuse among lesbian and bisexual women. Until recently, large-scale population-based studies of trauma rarely assessed for sexual orientation, and most assumed heterosexuality among participants (Balsam, 2003). Conversely, studies of lesbian, gay, and bisexual populations have generally not adequately assessed for trauma. In the past several years, researchers have begun to shed some light on this topic; the emerging picture suggests sexual minority women may experience elevated risk for interpersonal violence in both childhood (e.g., Corliss, Cochran & Mays, 2003; Tjaden, Thoeness, & Allison, 1999; Tomeo, Templer, Anderson, & Kotler, 2001) and adulthood (Balsam, 2002; Hughes, Johnson, & Wilsnak, 2001; Tjaden et al., 1999). In the current volume, the papers by D'Augelli, Robohm et al., Morris and Balsam, Cooperman et al., and Rose provide both quantitative and qualitative perspectives on the prevalence and nature of lesbian and bisexual women's experiences with victimization.

Developmental context plays a crucial role in understanding the impact of trauma. Two papers address this issue by providing empirical data from samples of adolescent and young adult women. D'Augelli's paper illustrates the prevalence of bias-related verbal, physical, and sexual victimization experiences among these young women and points to some of the factors that might mediate this risk. For example, earlier self-awareness and self-disclosure of sexual orientation was associated with even greater risk for bias-related victimization. This highlights one of the central dilemmas facing lesbian and bisexual youth. On the one hand, research with adult women has demonstrated that greater "outness" may positively impact mental health (e.g., Morris, Waldo, & Rothblum, 2001). On the other hand, when a young woman "comes out" she may be putting herself at greater risk; compared to an adult woman, she has relatively less control over her daily environment and may be forced to encounter discrimination, harassment, and violence in her home and school environment. Furthermore, D'Augelli found that worry about future victimization was a particularly strong predictor of mental health among these youths, pointing to the lack of safety these girls feel in their current environments. In their paper, Robohm, Litzenberger, and Pearlman take a closer look at the impact of sexual victimization on the lives of lesbian and bisexual youth. Similar to D'Augelli's results, these authors found that sexual abuse was associated with a wide array of self-reported emotional and behavioral difficulties.

The topic of childhood sexual abuse in the lives of sexual minority women is a particularly sensitive one, given the widespread myth in our culture that such abuse "causes" a person to become gay or lesbian. This "causality" hypothesis has been neither confirmed nor denied in the literature. Indeed, relatively few researchers have investigated the topic of sexual abuse among lesbian and bisexual women, perhaps out of fear of perpetuating myths and stereotypes. Two papers in this volume approach this issue but from a different angle. Rather than focusing on causality, the authors in this volume add to our understanding of the ways in which childhood sexual abuse impacts sexual identity development for women who come to identify as lesbian or bisexual. Robohm, Litzenberger, and Pearlman provide qualitative data to illustrate the range of ways in which young women make sense of their sexual abuse experiences. The quotes from individual women illustrate a range of ways in which these women understand the complex links between their abuse experiences and their processes of coming out as lesbian or bisexual. Morris and Balsam provide empirical data examining this relationship; their findings suggest that sexual abuse might indeed be associated with earlier awareness and identification of same-sex sexual attractions.

One of the major criticisms of sexual minority research to date has been the lack of heterogeneity among research samples. The "typical" sample includes women who are white and well-educated. The papers in this volume represent a shift towards greater inclusiveness and sensitivity to diversity than much of this previous literature. Several authors specifically focus on the experiences of sexual minority women of color. For example, Morris and Balsam report findings from a large national sample that includes a significant proportion of women of color. By comparing rates of victimization across ethnic groups, these authors found that certain groups of lesbian and bisexual women might experience even greater risk for victimization. This highlights the importance of recruiting large enough numbers of ethnic minority participants to make these comparisons. Cooperman, Simoni, and Lockhart report findings from a sample of predominantly African American and Latina women in New York City. Unlike previous samples of college-educated lesbians, participants in their study, on average, did not complete high school and were unemployed at the time of the study. Thus, this paper provides a valuable window into the lives of more marginalized women in the LGB community. Furthermore, Cooperman et al.'s sample consisted of HIV+ women, another group that has been largely neglected in studies of sexual minority women and victimization. Interestingly, sexual minority status was associated with greater risk for victimization in Cooperman et al.'s study, highlighting some similarities with previous studies.

Another theme of this volume is the intersection between trauma and oppression. In the current literature, definitions of trauma typically focus on a discrete event or events. For example, in the *Diagnostic and Statistical Manual, 4th edition* (*DSM-IV*; American Psychiatric Association, 1994), trauma is defined as "the personal experience of an event that involves actual or threatened death or serious injury, or other threat to one's physical integrity; or witnessing an event that involves death, injury, or a threat to the physical integrity of another person; or learning about unexpected or violent death, serious harm, or threat of death or injury experienced by a family member or other close associate" (p. 424).

The inclusion of the diagnosis Post-Traumatic Stress Disorder in the *DSM-III* (American Psychiatric Association, 1980) gave an official label to the psychological "fallout" of trauma. Importantly, this diagnosis was the first to make explicit the connection between external events and internal psychological distress. Thus, the study of traumatic stress represented a shift towards incorporating context into our understanding of human psychology. As the field of trauma studies has grown, increasing attention has been paid to broader contexts in which traumatic events occur. For example, interpersonal victimization has been highlighted as a specific subset of trauma, with the psychological impact being shaped by the interpersonal nature of the event (Finklehor & Kendall-Tackett, 1997). Response to traumatic events is also related to factors such as gender or ethnicity (Kimerling, Ouimette, & Wolfe, 2002; Marsella, Friedman, Gerrity, & Scurfield, 1996). Furthermore, contextual factors such as social support have been found to influence the process of recovery from trauma (Brewin, Andres, & Valentine, 2000).

Despite the emphasis on contextual factors, relatively little scholarship has focused on the context of homophobia in understanding experiences of trauma. A few authors have attempted to address this issue by broadening our understanding of the term "trauma." For example, Root (1992) makes the distinction between "direct traumas" such as physical and sexual abuse, "indirect traumas" that occurs when hearing or learning about direct traumas experienced by others, and "insidious trauma" experienced by members of oppressed group. She defines insidious trauma as the daily, ongoing stress associated with living with oppressions such as homophobia, sexism, or racism. Similarly, Neisen (1993) coined the term "cultural victimization" to refer to the impact of living in a heterosexist culture, and likens this experience to the trauma of physical and sexual abuse, explaining how both can lead to shame, negative self-concept, self-destructive behaviors, and a "victim mentality." Both of these models highlight the importance of examining the overlap between individual and cultural stressors. Looking closely at context, any direct trauma that takes place in the lives of lesbian and bisexual women must be understood against a backdrop of cultural or insidious trauma. The impact of these multiple traumas might interact in ways that look different than the impact of victimization in the lives of heterosexual individuals. For lesbian and bisexual women of color, this effect is magnified, as they experience the dual "cultural victimizations" of racism and heterosexism.

In the current volume, two papers focus specifically on the role of that "insidious traumas" play in the lives of lesbian and bisexual women. Bowleg, Huang, Brooks, Black, and Burkholder explore the intersections of sexism, racism, and homophobia in a sample of African American lesbians. The qualitative approach taken by these authors provides the opportunity to gain insights into the complexities of challenges facing this multiply marginalized group of women and provides rich examples of the meanings these women give to their experiences. Although women in this study gave personal examples of sexist and heterosexist experiences, racism was experienced as the most salient and meaningful stressor in their lives. Morrow's paper explores the nature and impact of religious oppression in the lives of lesbian and bisexual women, highlighting the intersection between cultural forces and individual experiences. For example, the author examines the struggles that some lesbians experience during the coming out process as they attempt to reconcile their religious beliefs with their emerging sexual feelings. She also examines how religious institutions have shaped the practice of conversion therapy, which in turn has harmed individual lesbians by promoting the internalization of shame and homophobic beliefs.

A final theme explored in this volume is that of resilience. In any study of marginalized groups, we run the risk of focusing too strongly on adversity and thereby viewing these individuals through the lens of pathology. While sexual minority women do, indeed, face many unique challenges and stressors, they also demonstrate unique strengths and resilience factors that are worthy of scholarly attention. Unlike heterosexuals, sexual minority women must learn to cope with "cultural victimization" on a daily basis. They must find a way to manage the conflict between their own feelings and societal norms. In pursuing same-sex relationships, they must confront the discrepancy between their own desires and the expectations of their families and communities. Throughout their lives, they must face the issue of whether and how much to self-disclose their identities in interactions with strangers, colleagues, and family members. As they negotiate these challenges, sexual minority women may develop a broader repertoire of coping skills that can then be utilized to manage the impact of other types of adversity.

Several papers in this volume address the issue of resilience. Both D'Augelli and Cooperman et al.'s studies highlight the importance of social support. In D'Augelli's paper, support and acceptance from both parents and friends played an important role in the mental health of young lesbian and bisexual women. In Cooperman et al.'s sample of HIV+ women, the lesbian and bisexual women reported greater HIV-related support than the heterosexual women. For all participants, social support was associated with lower depression, regardless of their history of victimization. Similarly, Bowleg et al.'s participants emphasize the importance of supportive relationships as strategies for managing the stresses associated with their marginalized identities. Morrow points out the importance of finding connection with others in the context of affirmative spiritual or religious organizations.

Another way that sexual minority women demonstrate resilience lies in the meanings and interpretations that they attach to their experiences. Bowleg et al.'s paper also highlights the importance of these internal strategies. For example, several of their participants focused on the "uniqueness" of being a Black lesbian, while others stated that they viewed this identity as a "gift." Others focused on the "freedom" or "liberation" that they experienced in being able to live according to their own desires, rather than following societal prescriptions for roles and relationships. Another crucial resilience strategy involves identifying and labeling sources of oppression; this strategy is addressed in both Morrow's and Bowleg et al.'s papers. Bowleg et al. also point out the importance of more direct strategies for dealing with oppression, such as directly confronting oppressive situations or refusing to allow others to define one's experiences.

In addition to examining resilience on the individual level, it is crucial to identify community-level approaches that promote resilience among sexual minority women. Rose's paper provides an excellent example of how researchers can form partnerships with community organizations to bring about change on a broader scale. Using data from a community survey focusing on bias-related crimes and same-sex domestic violence, as well as utilization data from an Anti-Violence Project (AVP) hotline, the author began to dialogue with local community organizations, law enforcement, and the media regarding the need for appropriate services to address these problems. In her paper, Rose provides specific case examples illustrating how homophobia shaped the nature, impact, and response to victimization experiences of lesbian and bisexual women who called the anti-violence hotline. She discusses how these case examples were useful in illustrating the need for services to community leaders and legislators. Rose describes how these dialogues resulted in community-level interventions to address violence against sexual minorities. For example, the Anti-Violence Project worked with the police and other community organizations to increase sensitivity and responsiveness to hate crimes and same-sex domestic violence. Furthermore, the AVP used their qualitative and quantitative data to advocate for legislative change, resulting in the passing of a Hate Crime Bill in the state of Missouri. Thus, by gathering information about the context of violence in the lives of sexual minorities, the author and her colleagues helped to enact changes that might ultimately improve that context.

In conclusion, it has been a great pleasure to edit this collection of interesting and important scholarly works. It is my sincere hope that this volume will provide a springboard from which researchers, clinicians, and activists can continue to dialogue about trauma, stress, and resilience in the sexual minority community. One of the parallels between trauma and oppression is the central role of silence in perpetuating shame and distress. In contrast, speaking out about trauma and oppression can build connections and foster healing. Speaking out is particularly important as the lesbian, gay, bisexual, and transgender community gains greater visibility. As with any oppressed group, we run the risk of believing that we must put forward an image of perfection, hiding our shortcomings from the public in order to continue to enjoy the benefits of social acceptance. While we have a great deal to be proud of, as with any community of people, we have our vulnerabilities as well. Armed with this knowledge, it is imperative that we continue to advocate for safety, justice, and healing within our families, communities, and society at large. Like the phoenix rising from the ashes, we can emerge from these challenges resilient, proud, and strong.

REFERENCES

American Psychiatric Association (1980). *Diagnostic and statistical manual of mental disorders* (3rd ed.). Washington, DC: Author.

American Psychiatric Association (1994). *Diagnostic and statistical manual of mental disorders* (4th ed.). Washington, DC: Author.

Balsam, K. F. (2002). *Traumatic victimization: A comparison of lesbian, gay, and bisexual adults and their heterosexual siblings*. Unpublished doctoral dissertation.

Balsam, K. F. (2003). Traumatic victimization in the lives of lesbian and bisexual women: A contextual approach. *Journal of Lesbian Studies, 7*(1), 1-14.

Brewin, C. R., Andrews, B., & Valentine, J. D. (2000). Meta-analysis of risk factors for posttraumatic stress disorder in trauma-exposed adults. *Journal of Consulting and Clinical Psychology, 68*, 748-766.

Corliss, H. L., Cochran, S. D., & Mays, V. M. (2002). Reports of parental maltreatment during childhood in a United States population-based survey of homosexual, bisexual, and heterosexual adults. *Child Abuse & Neglect, 26*, 1165-1178.

Finkelhor, D., & Kendall-Tackett, K. (1997). A developmental perspective on the childhood impact of crime, abuse, and violent victimization. In D. Cicchetti & S. L. Toth (Eds.), *Developmental perspectives on trauma: Theory, research, and intervention*. Rochester symposium on developmental psychology, Vol. 8 (pp. 1-32). Rochester, NY: University of Rochester Press.

Hughes, T. L., Johnson, T., & Wilsnack, S. C. (2001). Sexual assault and alcohol abuse: A comparison of lesbians and heterosexual women. *Journal of Substance Abuse, 13*, 515-532.

Kimerling, R., Ouimette, P., & Wolfe, J. (Eds.). (2002). *Gender and PTSD*. New York: Guilford.

Marsella, A. J., Friedman, M. J., Gerrity, E. T., & Scurfield, R. M. (1996). *Ethnocultural aspects of Posttraumatic Stress Disorder: Issues, research, and clinical applications*. Washington, D.C.: American Psychological Association.

Morris, J. F., Waldo, C. R., & Rothblum, E. D. (2001). A model of predictors and outcomes of outness among lesbian and bisexual women. *American Journal of Orthopsychiatry, 71*, 61-71.

Root, M. P. (1992). Reconstructing the impact of trauma on personality. In L.S. Brown & M. Ballou (Eds.), *Personality and psychopathology: Feminist reappraisals* (pp. 229-265). New York: Guilford.

Tjaden, P., Thoeness, N., & Allison, C. J. (1999). Comparing violence over the life span in samples of same-sex and opposite-sex cohabitants. *Violence and Victims, 14*(4), 413-425.

Tomeo, M. E., Templer, D. I., Anderson, S., & Kotler, D. (2001). Comparative data of childhood and adolescent molestation in heterosexual and homosexual persons. *Archives of Sexual Behavior, 30*, 535-541.

Lesbian and Bisexual Female Youths Aged 14 to 21: Developmental Challenges and Victimization Experiences

Anthony R. D'Augelli

SUMMARY. Two hundred six lesbian and bisexual female youth aged 14 to 21 were sampled from social and recreational settings. Most were aware of their same-sex attractions in adolescence, but disclosure to others lagged by five years. Youth on average spent 30% of their lives aware of their orientation without disclosure to others. According to youths' reports, three-quarters of their mothers and half of their fathers knew of

---

Anthony R. D'Augelli, PhD, is Professor of Human Development in the Department of Human Development and Family Studies at Penn State. He is a community psychologist whose primary research interests have concerned sexual orientation and human development in community settings. He has completed several research projects on lesbian, gay, and bisexual people, both adolescents and older adults who are 60 years of age or older. He is currently conducting a longitudinal study of the effects of victimization on the mental health of lesbian, gay, and bisexual youth.

Address correspondence to: Anthony R. D'Augelli, PhD, Department of Human Development and Family Studies, 105Q White Building, Pennsylvania State University, University Park, PA 16802 (E-mail: ard@psu.edu).

Completion of this report was facilitated by grant MH58155 from the National Institute of Mental Health.

[Haworth co-indexing entry note]: "Lesbian and Bisexual Female Youths Aged 14 to 21: Developmental Challenges and Victimization Experiences." D'Augelli, Anthony R. Co-published simultaneously in *Journal of Lesbian Studies* (Harrington Park Press, an imprint of The Haworth Press, Inc.) Vol. 7, No. 4, 2003, pp. 9-29; and: *Trauma, Stress, and Resilience Among Sexual Minority Women: Rising Like the Phoenix* (ed: Kimberly F. Balsam) Harrington Park Press, an imprint of The Haworth Press, Inc., 2003, pp. 9-29. Single or multiple copies of this article are available for a fee from The Haworth Document Delivery Service [1-800-HAWORTH, 9:00 a.m. - 5:00 p.m. (EST). E-mail address: docdelivery@haworthpress.com].

http://www.haworthpress.com/store/product.asp?sku=J155

10.1300/J155v07n04_02

their sexual orientation. Half had experienced repetitive verbal abuse, 12% reported several threats, and 7% had been assaulted multiple times. Youths who had self-identified as lesbian or bisexual or had told others of their sexual orientation reported more lifetime sexual orientation victimization. Fewer mental health symptoms were associated with having support from parents and with having not lost friends due to their sexual orientation. Less past sexual orientation victimization and fewer fears about future attacks were significant predictors of having less mental health symptoms. To decrease the victimization young lesbians and bisexual females experience, efforts need to be made to help families become more supportive and to make schools safer.

KEYWORDS. Sexual orientation, homosexuality, lesbians, youth, violence, victimization, harassment

Increasing attention has been directed toward the challenges and developmental pathways of lesbian and bisexual female youths, who have been studied much less often than gay and bisexual male youths (Schneider, 2001). There are only a handful of research reports that deal exclusively with lesbian and bisexual females under the age of 21. With the emergence of population-based studies of lesbian, gay, and bisexual youths during the 1990s (e.g., Remafedi, French, Story, Resnick, & Blum, 1998), more information about lesbian and bisexual youths has become available. For instance, Saewyc and her colleagues have conducted several population-based studies of health and mental health risk behavior of lesbian and bisexual adolescents (e.g., Saewyc, Bearinger, Heinz, Blum, & Resnick, 1998). Diamond (1998) demonstrated the variability of identity development patterns found among young females with same-sex sexual attractions. Research on young lesbian and bisexual females, however, does not often focus simultaneously on developmental and contextual factors that influence their adjustment. These youths' development cannot be well understood without an analysis of their social contexts–their families, their peer social networks, their school circumstances, and their communities. Specifically, the adolescent years are especially challenging for lesbian, gay, and bisexual youths because of the age at which they self-identify (a developmental factor) and because they are living at home and are in junior or senior high school (contextual factors). Of course, just as there are individual differences in the developmental processes leading to adult sexual identities, lesbian, gay, and bisexual youths differ substantially in the nature of the social contexts they contend with. Both the life stressors as well as the resources of lesbian, gay, and bisexual youths need to be identified to determine the nature of the relationship between these stressors, resources, and adjustment.

Using a diverse sample of lesbian and bisexual youths from 14 to 21 years of age, this report first presents information about the ages at which these youths reached a set of milestones associated with the development of their sexual orientation. Challenges faced at home and in school will then be noted, followed by experiences of victimization based on their sexual orientation. Their current adjustment–measured by self-esteem and reports of mental health symptoms–will be examined in light of challenges they face and social resources they have at their disposal.

Several general research questions guided analyses. It was expected that females who self-identified as lesbian or bisexual and had told others at earlier ages would likely experience more victimization than those who self-identified and self-disclosed later. Also, because of their ages, it was expected that more positive relationships with parents, and parents' knowledge of and positive reactions to their daughters' sexual orientation, would be associated with better adjustment. It was expected that relationships with mothers would be particularly important for youth's adjustment. Mother-adolescent daughter relationships can be very close, with mothers serving as important sources of support (Larson & Richards, 1994). Mothers have more daily contact with daughters than fathers, and are the socializing agents to whom young females often turn for advice about dating and sexual matters (Lefkowitz, Sigman, & Au, 2000). Mothers more so than fathers might feel that they failed in their parenting when a daughter comes out as lesbian or bisexual, and might experience more disappointment because of violation of traditional expectations that their daughters will marry and have families.

METHOD

Participants

Two data-sets were combined for these analyses. The first data were gathered from 1987 through 1989, and the second from 1995 to 1997. Similar data collection procedures were used both times. Letters were sent to adult coordinators of community groups for lesbian, gay, and bisexual young people across the United States and Canada, requesting that they consult with their group members about participation in the research. Groups interested in involvement were asked to notify the researcher. An adult contact person was identified in each group who served as liaison to the project. This person distributed the self-administered questionnaires in group meetings, and assured the researchers that human subjects requirements were met. Details about procedures can be found in D'Augelli and Hershberger (1993) and in D'Augelli, Hershberger, and Pilkington (2001).

The returned questionnaires included 542 youth who were 21 years of age or younger. Of these, 232 (43%) were female. Youths were asked to describe their sexual orientation using six categories: lesbian; bisexual, but mostly lesbian; bisexual, equally lesbian and heterosexual, bisexual, but mostly heterosexual, heterosexual, or uncertain. Youths who said they were bisexual, but mostly heterosexual (16), heterosexual (1), unsure (7), or who left the question blank (2) were excluded, resulting in a working sample of 206. This was done to create a more homogeneous sample of females whose sexual orientation was not more heterosexual than lesbian. Two-thirds (66%) identified as lesbian, and one-third as bisexual (34%; 21% said they were bisexual, but mostly lesbian and 13% said bisexual, but equally lesbian and heterosexual).

The 206 female respondents averaged 18.9 years of age ($SD = 1.55$); 15% were from 14 to 17; 48% were 18 or 19; and, 37% were either 20 or 21. Three-quarters (77%) were White; 7% were African American, 4% were of Hispanic origin, 2% were Native American or Canadian Indian, and the rest came from a variety of other backgrounds. Geographical diversity was reasonably represented: 35% lived in major metropolitan areas, 23% in small cities, 27% in medium-sized towns or in the suburbs, 10% in small towns, and 5% in rural areas. About one-third (37%) lived with their parents, 11% with partners, 16% with friends, and 14% in campus housing. Half (47%) reported they had a same-sex romantic partner. Of those with partners, 19% of the partners were the same age as the participants, 25% were younger (ranging from 1 to 3 years younger), and more than half (56%) were older (ranging from 1 to 11 years older).

Instrument

Sexual Orientation Development

Youths were asked about the ages at which important milestones related to the development of their sexual orientation occurred. Specifically, they were asked the age at which they were first aware of same-sex attraction, the age at which they first self-identified as lesbian or bisexual, the age of their first disclosure of same-sex attractions to another person, and the age at which they first told a parent they were lesbian or bisexual. Additional indicators of early sexual orientation experience were calculated. Years of awareness of lesbian and bisexual orientation were computed by subtracting youths' age at first awareness from their current age; years before self-identification was age of awareness subtracted from age of self-identification; and, years before first disclosure was the subtraction of age at self-identification from age of first disclosure. These scores reflect the duration of different phases of sexual orientation development. The percentage of youths' lives during which they were aware of same-sex feelings was calculated by dividing the age at which youths' reported their first awareness by their age. To approximate the percentage of their lives youths knew of their sexual orientation but had not told anyone, the difference between the age of self-identification and the age of first disclosure was divided by youths' age. Finally, as an indicator of the percentage of youths' lives spent self-identified as lesbian and bisexual but nondisclosed (perhaps the best indicator of time "in the closet" as they had labeled themselves), age of self-identification was subtracted from age of first disclosure, and then divided by youths' age. Relationships between milestones and disclosure to a parent were also examined. Of particular importance was how long youths had self-identified yet had not told their parents.

The participants were also asked when they had their first sexual experience with a female and with a male ("How old were you when you had your first sexual experience with a male/female?"). Finally, they estimated the number of female and male sexual partners they had during their lifetimes {"With how many same-sex/opposite-sex partners have you had sexual experiences?"). Ten response options were provided for these questions, ranging from 1 = "None" through 10 = "More than 50." These categories were treated like interval-level data in analyses.

Finally, youths were asked how open they were in general about their sexual orientation. They responded using a seven-point scale with two anchoring extremes, 1 = "Lesbian, gay, and bisexual identity hidden," through 7 = "Complete openness and honesty about lesbian, gay, and bisexual identity."

Relationships with Parents

Youth were asked about their relationships with their parents in general. The question was, "How do you get along with your parents now?" Youths responded separately for mothers and for fathers using five-point scales, with 1 = "Excellent," 2 = "Very well," 3 = "Well," 4 = "Not well," and 5 = "Poorly."

Parents' reactions to youths' sexual orientation were examined with two questions. First, mothers' and fathers' knowledge was determined using a four-point scale. Response options were: 1 = "Definitely knows, and we have talked about it," 2 = "Definitely knows, but we have never talked about it," 3 =

"Probably knows or suspects," and 4 = "Does not know or suspect." Youths then were asked how their mothers and their fathers reacted to knowing of their sexual orientation (or would react if they did not know). Responses were on a four-point scale, with: 1 = "Accepting (or it would not matter)," 2 = "Tolerant (but not accepting)," 3 = "Intolerant (but not rejecting)," and 4 = "Rejecting."

Relationship to the Lesbian, Gay, and Bisexual Community

Youth were asked two questions related to their involvement with the other lesbian, gay, and bisexual people. They were asked how many of their good friends were lesbian, gay, and bisexual, answered from 1 = "None," through 5 = "All." Then they were asked how often they attended lesbian, gay, and bisexual social events (parties, dinners, etc.), and how often these events were related to organized lesbian, gay, and bisexual groups. The first question was answered using six options, from 1 = "Never" through 6 = "Once a week or more." The question about the relative time these social events were associated with organized lesbian, gay, and bisexual groups was answered one scale from 1 = "None," through 5 = "All." These questions were designed to explore the degree to which these social resources might be associated with youths' adjustment.

Sexual Orientation Victimization

Lifetime victimization. Information about lifetime experiences of six types of victimization based on sexual orientation were available in both data-sets: verbal abuse, threats of physical attack, objects being thrown, assaults (being punched, kicked, or beaten), threats with weapons, and sexual assaults. The question was, "How often have you experienced the following because someone knew or assumed you were lesbian or bisexual?" Thus the question specifically focused on sexual orientation. They were not asked about other personal characteristics that may have provoked victimization, nor whether they thought their victimization was a result of being female. Respondents noted how often each type of victimization occurred using these categories: never, once, twice, or three or more times. A verbal victimization score was created by adding responses to items concerning verbal abuse and threats of physical attack. A physical victimization score was the sum of responses to questions about objects thrown, assaults, assaults with weapons, and sexual assaults. A total victimization score was computed by summing the scores for all types of victimization. To normalize the distributions of these scores, log 10 transformations were applied.

Youths were also asked if they had lost friends as a result of their sexual orientation. Although not direct victimization, rejection by friends for lesbian, gay, and bisexual youths can create considerable distress, especially if these friends disclose youths' sexual orientation to others.

Victimization by family members. Youths were asked whether particular family members had ever verbally abused them, threatened to hurt them, and actually hit them because of their sexual orientation. They were not asked about more specific types of verbal or physical abuse. These questions were answered for mothers, fathers, brothers, and sisters; response options were Yes or No.

Fears related to sexual orientation victimization. Youths were asked whether their current openness about their sexual orientation was influenced by fears of verbal or physical attacks. They were asked about the following: fear of losing friends, fear of being verbally abused at school, fear of being physically attacked at school, fear of being verbal abused at home, and fear of being physical attacked at home. Youths simply noted whether they had each fear. A total fear score was computed by adding the endorsements of these fears. They were asked whether they had reported incidents of harassment or violence to appropriate officials. They were also asked whether they had modified their behavior to avoid being attacked because of their sexual orientation, such as avoiding certain locations, or not walking with known lesbian, gay, and bisexual people.

Adjustment Indicators

Youths completed the Rosenberg Self-Esteem Inventory (RSEI; Rosenberg, 1979), and the Brief Symptom Inventory (BSI; Derogatis, 1993). The RSEI is a commonly-used measure of self-esteem; its Cronbach's alpha was .73 for the scores used here. The BSI is a standardized measure that asks the respondent to rate the occurrence and severity of 53 symptoms over the last two weeks. The BSI yields nine symptom subscales, but only a summary symptom score calculated by averaging the endorsement ratings of all symptoms, the Global Severity Index (GSI), was used in analyses. The BSI's reliability and validity are well-established, and Cronbach's alpha was .95 for GSI scores. The mean GSI score was used to account for missing data, and a log 10 transformation was used to normalize the distribution.

Information about more severe emotional distress was obtained by asking about past suicidal ideation and suicide attempts. Youths were first asked, "Have you *ever* seriously thought of taking your own life?" which was answered on a four-point scale ranging from 1 = "Never," through 4 = "Often." They were asked whether they had ever tried to kill themselves, answered as

Yes or No. Youths in the second study were asked more detailed questions about suicidality; results can be found in D'Augelli et al. (2001).

RESULTS

Sexual Orientation Development

Information about developmental milestones of youths' sexual orientation is shown in Table 1. Youths reported their first awareness of their same-sex

TABLE 1. Sexual Orientation Development Milestones of Lesbian and Bisexual Youths

Development Milestone	*n*	*M*	*SD*	Range
Age at First Awareness	205	11.10	4.07	2-19
Age at First Self-Identification	193	15.69	2.51	6-21
Age at First Disclosure	194	16.64	1.90	10-21
Age at First Disclosure to a Parent	151	17.26	2.11	8-21
Years of Awareness[a]	205	7.78	4.23	0-.17
Years Between Awareness and Self-Identification[b]	192	4.68	3.88	0-14
Years Between Self-Identification and Disclosure[c]	192	.96	1.78	0-14
Years Between Self-Identification and Disclosure to a Parent[d]	146	1.67	2.42	0-14
% of Life Aware[e]	192	.59	.22	.11-1
% of Life Aware but not Self-Identified[f]	192	.25	.20	0-.74
% of Life Aware but Non-Disclosed[g]	192	.30	.21	0-.78
% of Life Self-identified but Non-Disclosed[h]	192	.05	.09	−.06-.67
% of Life Self-identified but Not Disclosed to a Parent[i]	146	.09	.13	0-.67
Age at First Sexual Behavior with Males	151	13.17	3.80	3-21
Age at First Sexual Behavior with Females	181	15.86	3.24	5-21

[a]Age − Year of First Awareness
[b]Age at Self-Identification
[c]Age of First Disclosure − Age at Self-Identification
[d]Age of First Disclosure to a Parent − Age of Self-Identification
[e]Age of Awareness/Age
[f](Age of Self-Identification − Age of Awareness)/Age
[g](Age of First Disclosure − Age at First Awareness)/Age
[h](Age of First Disclosure − Age at Self-Identification)/Age
[i](Age of First Telling Parent − Age at Self-Identification)/Age

feelings at about age 11; self-identification occurred about five years later, at about 16. First disclosure of sexual orientation occurred at about 17, though youths reported this occurring as young as 10 years of age and as old as 21. Fourteen percent disclosed between the ages of 10 and 14; 69% between 15 and 18; and, 17% disclosed between 19 and 21. First disclosure to a parent, most often mothers, occurred at about the same time, at 17. Youths were aware of their same-sex feelings for about eight years, a little more than half of their lives. Youths spent about five years from the time they first became aware of their sexual feelings and when they self-identified. They spent 30% of their lives aware of their sexual orientation without telling anyone. There was wide variability in the time youths spent "in the closet," ranging from under one year (disclosure occurred in the same year as awareness) to over 80% of youths' lives. If one uses age of self-identification as the marker against which to compare age of first disclosure, youths were found to have spent about 7% of their lives self-identified yet nondisclosed. Clearly the largest amount of time is spent between awareness and disclosure; disclosure follows self-identification much more rapidly.

Most (196 youths or 95%) reported that they had had sexual experience with either a male or a female, and 136 (69%) reported that they had had sex with both male and female partners. One hundred and eighty-one (88%) reported having had a female sexual partner, and 12% had not. The average age of initiation of sexual behavior with another female was 16, and the range was from 5 to 21. As to male partners, three-quarters (151) had had sexual contact with a male, with an average age of initiation of 13, with a range of from 3 to 21. Most who reported female and male sexual partners experienced sex with a male partner first. In 77% of the cases, age of first sex with males preceded age of first sex with females; in 8% these events occurred at the same age; and, 15% had sex with a female before sex with a male. This difference might reflect more unwanted sex from males at earlier ages, perhaps even childhood sexual abuse, but the nature of the first sexual experiences (were they voluntary or coerced) was not asked. Table 2 shows the frequencies of female and male sexual partners reported.

As to openness about their sexual orientation, the average openness score was 5.23 (SD = 1.60), above the midpoint on the scale. About one-quarter (24%) endorsed the highest openness score, whereas 3% said they were completely hidden. Only 15% scored below the midpoint of the scale, and 71% scored above the midpoint.

Relationship to Parents

Over one-quarter of the participants said that relationships with fathers were excellent; more (42%) rated relationships with their mothers as excellent.

TABLE 2. Number of Same-Sex and Opposite-Sex Sexual Partners of Lesbian and Bisexual Youths

Number of Sexual Partners	Same-Sex		Opposite-Sex	
	n	%	*n*	%
None	20	10	51	26
1	35	17	25	13
2-4	96	47	62	31
5-7	29	14	25	13
8-10	11	5	9	5
11-13	5	2	11	6
14-19	3	1	6	3
20-30	0	0	5	2
31-50	0	0	1	< 1
51+	3	1	1	< 1

For same-sex partners $n = 202$; for opposite-sex partners $n = 196$.

At the other extreme of the ratings, 29% of the youths said they did not get along well with their fathers, and 34% evaluated their relationships with mothers in the same way. No difference between ratings of relationships with mothers and fathers was found, and ratings of parents were significantly correlated, $r\,(164) = .31, p < .001$.

Table 3 presents youths' reports of parents' knowledge of their daughters' sexual orientation, and their reactions (or predicted reactions for parents who did not know). More mothers were aware of youths' sexual orientation. Nearly three-quarters of the mothers, compared to about half of the fathers, knew about and had discussed the issue. Nearly one-quarter of the fathers were thought to not know or suspect, compared to 10% of the mothers. Mothers' were viewed as significantly more knowledgeable, $t\,(171) = 5.87, p < .001$. One-quarter of mothers (26%) and more than one-third (37%) of fathers were labeled either intolerant or rejecting of their daughters' sexual orientation; at the most positive end of the rating, half (49%) of mothers and one-third (37%) of fathers were accepting. Thus, half of the mothers and two-thirds of the fathers were considered less than fully accepting. Fathers were significantly less accepting, $t\,(157) = 2.77, p < .01$.

A correlation matrix was produced relating ratings of relationships with parents, parents' knowledge, and parents' reactions. Knowledge of youths' sexual orientation was unrelated to the youths' reports of how well they related

TABLE 3. Parents' Knowledge of and Reactions to Their Daughters' Sexual Orientation

	Knowledge								Reaction							
Parent	Knows, Have Talked		Knows, No Talk		Suspects		Doesn't Know		Accepting		Tolerant		Intolerant		Rejecting	
	n	%	*n*	%	*n*	%	*n*	%	*n*	%	*n*	%	*n*	%	*n*	%
Mother	135	71	17	9	20	10	19	10	88	49	45	25	17	9	30	17
Father	86	49	31	18	17	10	41	23	59	37	42	26	27	17	31	20

to their parents, but strong relationships emerged with parental reactions. More positive mothers' reactions, $r\,(169) = .44$, $p < .001$, and more positive fathers' reactions, $r\,(149) = .43$, $p < .001$, were significantly associated with better relationships.

Relationship to the Lesbian, Gay, and Bisexual Community

Many youths' best friends were lesbian, gay, and bisexual. Five percent said all their best friends were lesbian, gay, and bisexual, 48% said more than half, 24% said half, 22% said less than half, and 1% said none. As to attendance at lesbian, gay, and bisexual social events, nearly one-third (31%) said they attended such events at least weekly; 10% said monthly; and, 24% said five times a year or less. Similar variability was also seen in social activity with members of lesbian, gay, and bisexual organized groups: 11% said none of their socializing was with such groups or their members, 25% said less than half, 17% said half, 29% said more than half, and 19% said all of their activities were with group members. Thus, despite being sampled in social and recreational groups for lesbian, gay, and bisexual youths, much of their socializing was with others.

Sexual Orientation Victimization

Lifetime victimization. Table 4 shows lifetime victimization based on their sexual orientation. Over the course of their lives, 75% of participants have been verbally abused, 30% have been threatened with physical attack, 17% have had objects thrown at them, 13% have been physically assaulted, 4% have been assaulted with a weapon, and 12% have been sexually assaulted. Many youths reported multiple incidents of victimization. Half (51%) had been subjected to three or more incidents of verbal abuse, 12% had been threatened with violence three or more times, and 7% had been physically attacked three or more times because of their sexual orientation. Unfortunately, the ages at which these events first occurred were not sought, so it is unknown whether they occurred when participants were children or adolescents.

As predicted, there was a significant relationship between the age of self-identification as lesbian or bisexual and sexual orientation victimization. Participants who self identified earlier reported more lifetime sexual orientation victimization, $r\,(166) = -.26$, $p < .001$, and those who disclosed to others when they were younger also reported more lifetime victimization, $r\,(166) = -.25$, $p < .001$. Similar results were obtained when sexual orientation milestone ages were correlated with both lifetime verbal victimization and lifetime physical victimization. Unfortunately, data about the ages at which victimiza-

TABLE 4. Lifetime Sexual Orientation Victimization of Lesbian and Bisexual Youths

Type	Never		Once		Twice		3+ Times	
	n	%	*n*	%	*n*	%	*n*	%
Verbal abuse (*n* = 189)	47	25	25	13	21	11	96	51
Threat of violence (*n* = 186)	131	70	19	10	14	8	22	12
Objects thrown (*n* = 187)	155	83	15	8	7	4	10	5
Assault (*n* = 188)	164	87	7	4	3	2	14	7
Threatened with weapon (*n* = 191)	183	96	3	2	2	1	3	2
Sexual assault (*n* = 191)	168	88	16	8	3	2	4	2

tion of different kinds occurred was not available. Thus, some of the victimization reported could have happened in childhood.

Victimization by family members. Verbal abuse by mothers was reported by 14% of the sample; 2% of mothers threatened their daughters; and, 7% hit them due to their sexual orientation. Victimization from fathers was less frequent, perhaps because fewer fathers knew about their daughters' sexual orientation. Only 4% of fathers verbally abused their daughters, 2% threatened them, and 2% hit them. Twelve youths reported that their brothers verbally abused them and six reported verbal abuse from sisters.

Fears related to sexual orientation. The following percentages of the sample reported experiencing specific fears related to their sexual orientation: fear of losing friends: 46% (89/195); fear of verbal abuse at school: 42% (81/192); fear of physical abuse at school: 28% (54/193); fear of verbal abuse at home: 35% (68/194); and, fear of physical abuse at home: 15% (29/192). Their fears of future victimization may help to account for the low rate of reporting victimization based on their sexual orientation to others. More than one-third (37%) did not report victimization they experienced to others, 40% reported some victimization experiences, and 22% reported every incident. More than one-third (39%) said they modified their behavior to avoid victimization.

Adjustment Indicators

Correlations were run to determine the independence of the adjustment indicators. More mental health symptoms as shown by higher GSI scores were associated with less self-esteem, $r\,(187) = -.48$, $p < .001$, and with more lifetime suicidal ideation, $r\,(185) = .45$, $p < .001$. Although these correlations are statistically significant, their magnitude indicates that the scores are not measuring the same construct, so they all were maintained in analyses. Of the sample, 15% (31) of the females said they often had serious thoughts about killing themselves, 27% (55) sometimes had these thoughts, 27% (54) rarely had such thoughts, and 31% (63) never had these thoughts. Suicide attempts were reported by 39% (77) of the sample.

Relationship of Sexual Orientation Victimization and Other Variables to Adjustment Indicators

Table 5 shows correlations between selected sexual orientation development milestones, relationships with parents, questions about youths' relationship to the lesbian, gay, and bisexual community, victimization histories, and the adjustment indicators–self-esteem, GSI scores, and suicidal ideation. Sexual orientation milestones were not related to either self-esteem or mental health symptoms. However, participants who were younger when they first be-

TABLE 5. Correlations of Major Variables with Mental Health Indicators

Variable	Self-Esteem	Overall Symptoms	Suicidal Ideation
Age	.05	−.12	−.07
Age at First Awareness	.08	−.11	−.16*
% of Life Aware	.07	−.08	−.15*
Age of First Sexual Behavior with Males	.03	−.16	−.22**
Age of First Sexual Behavior with Females	.07	−.13	−.07
Number of Male Sexual Partners	.08	.07	.14
Number of Female Sexual Partners	.21**	−.06	−.04
Mother's Knowledge of SO	−.11	.12	.03
Fathers's Knowledge of SO	−.08	.09	−.04
Mother's Reaction to SO	−.09	.19**	.09
Father's Reaction to SO	−.08	.09	.10
Involvement with Lesbian, Gay, and Bisexual Community	.09	.05	.12
Verbal SO Victimization	.07	.21**	.13
Physical SO Victimization	.14	.14*	.09
Total SO Victimization	.13	.21**	.13
Fears Related to SO Victimization	−.22**	.25**	.25**

Note. SO = Sexual Orientation; Overall Symptoms = log transformed mean Brief Symptom Inventory Global Severity Index score.
$^{*}p < .05$. $^{**}p < .01$.

came aware of their sexual orientation had more suicidal ideation. Females who were aware for more of their lives demonstrated less suicidal ideation. Youths with more suicidal ideation also reported having had sexual contact with a male at earlier ages. Higher self-esteem was associated with more same-sex sexual partners and fewer fears related to future victimization based on sexual orientation. The more negative mothers' reactions were to the youth, the more symptoms they reported. The more negative mothers were about their daughters' sexual orientation, the more symptoms youth reported. Higher victimization was related to more symptoms. As to suicidal ideation, earlier age of heterosexual sexual behavior and more fear of future victimization were related to more suicidal thinking. It must be noted that none of these correlations are substantial, with the largest accounting for only 6% of the variance involved.

Additional analyses were conducted to explore sources of support. Presuming that having parents who know and are positive about one's sexual orientation constitutes a positive source of support, three awareness groups were created: both parents knew, neither knew, or one knew and the other did not know. For approval, either both parents were accepting, both were not accepting, or one was accepting and one was not. Separate one-way analyses of variances were conducted using the three adjustment indicators as dependent variables, and significant results were followed up with Tukey tests (at $p < .05$). Overall mental health symptoms (GSI scores) were related to parental knowledge or support. For parental knowledge, having two knowledgeable parents was associated with fewer symptoms than having two parents who did not know, $F\ (2, 180) = 4.15, p < .05$. For parental reactions, exploration of the overall significant finding, $F\ (2, 172) = 3.39, p < .05$, showed that having two positive parents was related to less symptoms than having two negative parents. Suicide attempts were highest among youths with parents who did not know (23%).

Compared to youths who had lost friends as a result of their sexual orientation, youths who had not had significantly higher self-esteem, $t\ (197) = 3.00, p < .01$, lower overall symptom scores, $t\ (181) = 2.41, p < .05$, and less suicidal ideation, $t\ (195) = 7.99, p < .01$. Loss of friends was strongly associated with past suicide attempts. Of those who had lost friends, 57% reported a past attempt, compared to 42% who had not lost friends, $\chi^2\ (1) = 8.67, p < .001$.

Another support variable was created by combining parental reactions and loss of friends. Having supportive parents and not having lost friends were predicted to be associated with better adjustment than having negative parental reactions and having lost friends. Two categories were constructed. High Support youths had parents who were accepting, with no loss of friends; and,

Low Support youths had two negative parents and had lost friends. There were 68 youths (33%) in the High Support category, and 21 youths (10%) in the Low Support category. (The remainder of the youths had varied parental support and friendship experiences.) Because of the small number of Low Support youths, results should be considered with caution. The High and Low Support youths did not differ in self-esteem, but significant differences on the other adjustment measures were found. Youths with low support had significantly more mental health symptoms than youths with high support, t (84) = 2.75, $p < .01$. While no differences in lifetime suicidal ideation were found, significantly more Low Support youths (67% or 14/21) than High Support youths (34% or 23/68) reported a past suicide attempt, $\chi2$ (N = 89, df = 1) = 7.13, $p < .01$.

Finally, multiple regression analyses were conducted to determine which variables best predicted youths' mental health symptoms (GSI scores). Table 6 shows the results of a regression analysis using all of the variables in Table 5. These variables accounted for 16% (adjusted R^2) of the overall variance of the GSI scores. More sexual orientation victimization and more fear of future victimization predicted to more mental health symptoms. Thus, the most powerful influences on youths' current distress were amount of sexual orientation

TABLE 6. Predictors of Mental Health Symptoms

Variable	∃	*SE*	*t*
Age	.06	.09	.17
Age of First Awareness	−1.74	.13	−1.12
% of Life Aware	1.69	2.57	1.08
Number of Male Sexual Partners	.02	.03	.20
Number of Female Sexual Partners	.01	.05	.12
Age at First Sexual Behavior with a Male	−.12	.01	−.83
Age at First Sexual Behavior with a Female	.07	.02	.49
Mother's Knowledge of SO	.12	.06	.73
Father's Knowledge of SO	−.07	.05	−.46
Mother's Reaction to SO	−.14	.05	−.95
Father's Reaction to SO	.04	.04	.27
Involvement with Lesbian, Gay, and Bisexual Community	.03	.02	.26
Total SO Victimization	.27	.15	2.00*
Fears Related to SO Victimization	.36	.03	3.37**

Note: SO = Sexual Orientation
R^2 = .16, F (14, 69) = 2.09, $p < .05$.
*$p < .05$, ** $p < .01$.

victimization they had already experienced and fears about future victimization at home and in school.

DISCUSSION

These findings demonstrate the challenges faced by young females who identify as lesbian or bisexual during adolescence. Many of the participants in the study were aware of their feelings for other females late in their childhood years or in early adolescence. It would take several years for these feelings to be shared with others, and their disclosures generally followed relatively quickly after they self-identified as lesbian or bisexual. Disclosure to parents occurred somewhat later. Youths had spent about one-third of their lives aware of their sexual orientation without discussing it with others, a substantial, and unique, developmental period that heterosexual youths do not experience. As adolescence proceeds, more female youths become aware of the nature of their feelings, and have the cognitive, emotional, and social resources to cope with them. How they handle the process of disclosure–when, to whom, and under what conditions–can make a substantial difference in how they live their adolescent years. For instance, a young girl who at age 14 tells a supportive mother that she thinks she is bisexual, starts dating other girls, and spends more time with other lesbian and bisexual youths is on a very different developmental pathway than a 14-year-old with two highly disapproving parents, who repetitively express disdain for their daughter's "lifestyle," badger her into heterosexual dating, and make their disappointments with her clear for the years she remains at home.

Many of the youths–fully one-third–identified as bisexual, a higher proportion than seen among the gay and bisexual males represented in these data sets (D'Augelli, 2002). Nearly three-quarters of the females had sexual contact with a male, with heterosexual sexual contact often preceding same-sex sexual contact. Why females engage in more heterosexual behavior and identify more as bisexual could be a reflection of greater pressures to engage in traditional dating, the greater fluidity of female sexual orientation development, less rigid gender concepts, and less stigma associated with same-sex affection among females. Certainly some of these heterosexual experiences were coercive and nonconsensual, although this cannot be determined by these data, a weakness of the study. Another important factor is the lower visibility of lesbians in society, and the greater latitude allotted to women to express emotional and physical affection for other women. The latter processes might slow down identification as lesbian, and it may well be that the onset of sexual behavior with other females is a crucial step for bisexually-identified youths to move to lesbian identification. Schneider (2001), for example, found many differences among young females as to what constituted a "milestone," and has noted that the extra pressures that young females are under to conform to others' expectations may make it more difficult to take the steps needed to explore a lesbian identity. Another interesting issue relates to the role of relationship development in young lesbian identity development. It may well be that the social prohibitions placed on high school females to date females interferes with the development of their identities as lesbian; the lack of same-sex dating possibilities for males, though certainly important, may be less central to their identification as gay.

Disclosure of a lesbian or bisexual orientation during adolescence and young adulthood is contingent not only on developmental processes, but also on the social support youths have from families and friends (D'Augelli, Hershberger, & Pilkington, 1998). If having supportive families and experiencing little social censure or sexual orientation victimization facilitate socialization into an adult bisexual or lesbian identity status, having hostile families and being victimized because one is known to be lesbian or bisexual can produce stress, fear, and mental health problems, thus interfering with identity integration. The family stressors in these youths' lives are clear when their relationships with parents are examined. More mothers than fathers knew their daughters were lesbian or bisexual; importantly, more mothers were accepting. Parental reactions to sexual orientation related to youths' overall evaluation of their relationship to their parents. Having two parents who knew of their daughter's sexual orientation was associated with fewer mental health symptoms compared to having parents who were unaware. The importance of friends is also apparent. Youths who had lost friends specifically because of their sexual orientation had lower self-esteem and more mental health problems. The combination of unsupportive parents and the loss of friends is particularly difficult, and youths in this situation were particularly symptomatic. The loss of friends can have a cascading negative effect. For example, losing friends can increase distress in school as knowledge of youths' sexual orientation becomes known when rejecting friends tell others. The power of parents' and friends' reactions can also be seen in the suicide attempt results. Youths who had neither parent's support and had lost friends were found to have made efforts to end their lives. Given the correlational nature of these data, however, it is also possible that distressed youth alienate parents and friends, with the resultant isolation leading to suicide attempts.

Support from others is particularly important in light of the sexual orientation victimization that youths report, because such support can help to buffer the deleterious effects of such attacks (Hershberger & D'Augelli, 1995). Most youths had experienced verbal abuse; many had been threatened with physical attacks; and, some had been assaulted. The earlier youth had self-identified as bisexual or lesbian, the more lifetime sexual orientation victimization she reported, and the earlier youth had disclosed their sexual orientation, the more attacks they experienced. Some verbal abuse within the family was found, especially from mothers, perhaps because more mothers knew of their daughters' sexual orientation. What emerged as most important in terms of mental health, however, was a fear of future victimization, both at school and at home. Nearly half worried about losing more friends, and many were afraid that they would be verbally or physically hurt at school. Less fear about untoward events at home was seen, yet over one-third feared verbal abuse at home. Although the amount of victimization youths experienced predicted current mental health symptoms, it was fear of future attacks that was the most powerful correlate of symptoms. Other results from the second study whose data were used in these analyses revealed that half the youths reported verbal abuse in high schools, and 11% said they had been physically assaulted in schools (D'Augelli, Pilkington, & Hershberger, 2002). Youths who were more open in high school about their sexual orientation were victimized more, echoing the finding noted above that earlier disclosure was associated with more victimization. The amount of school-based victimization can help explain why so many participants feared verbal and physical abuse in school. It is also possible that the observation of what happens to "out" lesbian, gay, and bisexual youths in school serves to inhibit the expression of one's sexual orientation. The developmental impact over the lifespan of observing the victimization of other lesbian, gay, and bisexual people deserves further study, especially during adolescence.

For these young females, worry about being verbally abused or physically attacked can be a chronic stress lasting years, given that the time youths spend, in school-related activities, and at home. Surely some of the worry is also related to fears of being victimized as females. The social contexts of schools and families are of utmost importance in the lives of most adolescents, and this is no less true for lesbian, gay, and bisexual youths. The added burden of uncertain acceptance both with family and with peers leads many youths to hide their sexual orientation until early adulthood, when they are independent of families and are no longer in school. Increasing support from families can be encouraged by helping families dealing with conflicts about their children's sexual orientation. A complementary strategy would be to make schools safe for lgb students, and to establish sanctions for victimization based on actual or presumed sexual orientation.

There are several limitations of the study that deserve noting. The sample contains self-selected samples of lesbian and bisexual females who might not be representative of all young females with same-sex attractions. They are, on the other hand, likely representative of the young females who are sufficiently certain open about their sexual orientation to attend groups for lesbian, gay, and bisexual youth. Also, the data are self-reports, which have inherent difficulties. In this study, the issue of the accuracy of youths' attributions of the reasons they had been victimized is especially important, given the evidence that even lesbian, gay, and bisexual adult hate crime victims have difficulties disentangling the precipitants of their attacks, especially in ambiguous circumstances (Herek, Cogan, & Gillis, 2002). The cross-sectional nature of the data is another limitation, in that causality cannot be established. While it may seem much more probable that victimization is more likely to lead to adjustment difficulties than such difficulties would induce victimization, such conclusions required longitudinal data.

Despite the limitations of the study, the evidence of the challenges faced by young lesbians and bisexual females requires the attention of professionals who work with youth. As increasing numbers of adolescents come out at earlier ages, families and schools are the crucial social contexts that influence how well these youths make a successful transition to adulthood. The situation is especially urgent for younger adolescents who may not yet identify as lesbian or bisexual, but who experience same-sex sexual and emotional attractions. Developing ways to help families understand and accept their lesbian and bisexual daughters and implementing procedures and policies to prevent victimization based on sexual orientation are required if future difficulties among this population are to be decreased.

REFERENCES

D'Augelli, A. R. (2002). Mental health problems among lesbian, gay, and bisexual youths ages 14 to 21. *Clinical Child Psychology and Psychiatry, 7*, 439-462.

D'Augelli, A. R., & Hershberger, S. L. (1993). Lesbian, gay, and bisexual youth in community settings: Personal challenges and mental health problems. *American Journal of Community Psychology, 21*, 421-448.

D'Augelli, A. R., Hershberger, S. L., & Pilkington, N. W. (1998). Lesbian, gay, and bisexual youths and their families: Disclosure of sexual orientation and its consequences. *American Journal of Orthopsychiatry, 68*, 361-371.

D'Augelli, A. R., Hershberger, S. L., & Pilkington, N. W. (2001). Suicidality patterns and sexual orientation-related factors among lesbian, gay and bisexual youths. *Suicide and Life-Threatening Behavior, 31*, 250-265.

D'Augelli, A. R., Pilkington, N. W., & Hershberger, S. L. (2002). Incidence and mental health impact of sexual orientation victimization of lesbian, gay, and bisexual youths in high school. *School Psychology Quarterly, 17*, 148-167.

Derogatis, L. R. (1993). *The Brief Symptom Inventory: Administration, scoring, and procedures manual*. Minneapolis: National Computer Systems.

Diamond, L. M. (1998). Development of sexual orientation among adolescent and adult young women. *Developmental Psychology, 34*, 1085-1095.

Herek, G. M., Cogan, J. C., & Gillis, J. R. (2002). Victim experiences of hate crimes based on sexual orientation. *Journal of Social Issues, 58*(2), 319-339.

Hershberger, S. L., & D'Augelli, A. R. (1995). The impact of victimization on the mental health and suicidality of lesbian, gay, and bisexual youth. *Developmental Psychology, 31*, 65-74.

Larson, R. & Richards, M. (1994). Family emotions: Do adolescents and their parents experience the same states? *Journal of Adolescent Research, 4*, 567-583.

Lefkowitz, E. S., Sigman, M. D., & Au, T. K. (2000). Helping mothers discuss sexuality and AIDS with adolescents. *Child Development, 71*, 1384-1394.

Remafedi, G., French, S., Story, M., Resnick, M. D., & Blum, R. (1998). The relationship between suicide risk and sexual orientation: Results of a population-based survey. *American Journal of Public Health, 88*, 57-60.

Rosenberg, M. (1979). *Conceiving the self.* NY: Basic Books.

Saewyc, E. M., Bearinger, L. H., Heinz, P. A., Blum, R. W., & Resnick, M. D. (1998). Gender differences in health and risk behaviors among bisexual and homosexual adolescents. *Journal of Adolescent Health, 23*, 181-188.

Schneider, M. S. (2001). Toward a reconceptualization of the coming-out process for adolescent females. In A. R. D'Augelli & C. J. Patterson (Eds.), *Lesbian, gay, and bisexual identities and youth: Psychological perspectives* (pp. 71-96). New York: Oxford University Press.

Sexual Abuse in Lesbian and Bisexual Young Women: Associations with Emotional/Behavioral Difficulties, Feelings About Sexuality, and the "Coming Out" Process

Jennifer S. Robohm
Brian W. Litzenberger
Laurie Anne Pearlman

Jennifer S. Robohm and Brian W. Litzenberger were post-doctoral fellows at the Traumatic Stress Institute/Center for Adult & Adolescent Psychotherapy$_{LLC}$ (TSI/CAAP) in South Windsor, Connecticut, from 1997-1999. Jennifer S. Robohm, PhD, is now a clinical psychologist at Furman Counseling Center, Barnard College, New York, NY. Brian Litzenberger, PhD, is now in private practice in Worcester, MA.

Laurie Anne Pearlman, PhD, is Research Director at TSI/CAAP and President of the Trauma Research, Education, and Training Institute, Inc. (TREATI).

Address correspondence to: Jennifer S. Robohm, PhD, Furman Counseling Center, Barnard College, 3009 Broadway, New York, NY 10027-6598 (E-mail: jrobohm@barnard.edu).

The authors would like to thank Beth Tabor Lev, Sarah Nicholls, Linda Chapman, and Ronni Sanlo for their review of prior manuscripts, their assistance with research and technological aspects of the study, and their help in publicizing the questionnaire. The authors also extend sincere thanks to the many participants who volunteered their time and thoughts for this study.

[Haworth co-indexing entry note]: "Sexual Abuse in Lesbian and Bisexual Young Women: Associations with Emotional/Behavioral Difficulties, Feelings About Sexuality, and the 'Coming Out' Process." Robohm, Jennifer S., Brian W. Litzenberger, and Laurie Anne Pearlman. Co-published simultaneously in *Journal of Lesbian Studies* (Harrington Park Press, an imprint of The Haworth Press, Inc.) Vol. 7, No. 4, 2003, pp. 31-47; and: *Trauma, Stress, and Resilience Among Sexual Minority Women: Rising Like the Phoenix* (ed: Kimberly F. Balsam) Harrington Park Press, an imprint of The Haworth Press, Inc., 2003, pp. 31-47. Single or multiple copies of this article are available for a fee from The Haworth Document Delivery Service [1-800-HAWORTH, 9:00 a.m. - 5:00 p.m. (EST). E-mail address: docdelivery@haworthpress.com].

http://www.haworthpress.com/store/product.asp?sku=J155

10.1300/J155v07n04_03

SUMMARY. We examined associations between childhood sexual abuse (CSA) and emotional/behavioral difficulties, feelings about one's sexuality, and the "coming out" process in a sample of 227 lesbian and bisexual women, ages 18-23, recruited for an online questionnaire study. Participants with a CSA history ("experiencers") reported significantly more emotional/behavioral difficulties than their nonexperiencer counterparts, suggesting that CSA may be an important contributor to some problems and behaviors currently linked in the literature to sexual orientation. Lesbian and bisexual experiencers varied widely as to whether and how they felt a CSA history affected their feelings about their sexuality or their "coming out" process. We discuss the implications of these findings for counseling, research, and theorizing involving lesbian and bisexual young women.

KEYWORDS. Sexual abuse, sexual assault, lesbian, bisexual, emotional/behavioral difficulties, sexuality, "coming out" process

In recent years, the needs of lesbian, gay, and bisexual (LGB) adolescents have received growing attention. Prior research has indicated that these youth may be at risk for a number of difficulties, including anxiety and depression, social isolation, running away, school problems, prostitution, alcohol/substance abuse, suicidality and self-injury, trouble with the law, and infection with HIV or other sexually transmitted diseases (Anhalt & Morris, 1998; Dempsey, 1994; Gibson, 1989; Lock & Steiner, 1999; Remafedi, 1987; Rotheram-Borus, Rosario, Meyer-Bahlburg, Koopman, Dopkins, & Davies, 1994; Savin-Williams, 1994). It has been suggested that factors related to being a sexual minority in a homophobic culture may explain the problems seen in this population (DiPlacido, 1998; Savin-Williams, 1994). It is reasonable to assume that other risk factors may also account for some of the distress seen in LGB youth.

Interestingly, there is a significant overlap between the problems reported for some LGB adolescents and the symptoms exhibited by many experiencers of childhood sexual abuse (CSA) and assault (e.g., Neumann, Houskamp, Pollack, & Briere, 1996). This overlap raises two possibilities worthy of empirical exploration. First, a significant number of LGB adolescents may be CSA experiencers, and some of the symptoms or difficulties exhibited by these youth (and commonly attributed to sexual orientation or the "coming out" process) may, in fact, be better attributed to experiences of childhood trauma. Second, for some LGB adolescents, their experience of their sexuality or their "coming out" process may be complicated or exacerbated by CSA experiences.

Why might we expect a connection, either direct or indirect, between LGB identification, behavioral/emotional problems, and CSA in some of these youth? Both a minority sexual orientation and sexual abuse involve sexual feelings which can feel confusing and can carry a sense of societal stigma or shame. Finkelhor and Browne (1985) argued that survivors of sexual abuse experience "traumatic sexualization" by which their sexuality is shaped in a developmentally inappropriate fashion, and they emerge from their experiences with "inappropriate repertoires of sexual behavior, with confusions and misconceptions about their sexual self-concepts, and with unusual emotional associations to sexual activities" (p. 531). Certainly, it is possible that an adolescent already struggling with such a sexualized self-concept and a stigmatized identity might then have particular difficulty when also wrestling with questions of sexual orientation in a homophobic society, causing him or her to experience emotional/behavioral problems.

It has also been suggested that sexual abuse may influence the process of sexual identity formation (Bartholow, Doll, Joy, Douglas, Bolan, Harrison, Moss, & McKirnan, 1994). For example, sexual abuse might impact psychosexual development, awareness of sexual orientation, and/or choice of sexual behavior. Further, because many gay youths engage in sexual activity as a means of exploring their sexual orientation (Rotheram-Borus, Rosario, Van Rossem, Reid, & Gillis, 1995), sexual abuse might also affect the timing of the "coming out" process. Specifically, some adolescents who had experienced CSA might engage in sexual activity sooner than their nonexperiencer peers, whereas others might delay or avoid sexual activity altogether. Both of these potential pathways might then have implications for LGB youth in terms of the formation and consolidation of their sexual identities and self-concepts.

A few studies have already indicated that adult gay and bisexual males with histories of CSA are more likely than those without such histories to report mental health counseling and hospitalization, substance use, depression, suicidal thoughts or actions, risky sexual behavior, and prostitution (Bartholow et al., 1994; Carballo-Dieguez & Dolezal, 1995; Lenderking, Wold, Mayer, Goldstein, Losina, & Seage, 1997). Further, a study of gay and bisexual males, ages 14-21, found that those who had attempted suicide were more likely to report sexual abuse than those who had not attempted suicide (Remafedi, Farrow, & Deisher, 1993).

Only a few studies have looked specifically at the emotional/behavioral impact of CSA on lesbian and bisexual women. Bradford, Ryan, and Rothblum (1994) measured the prevalence of physical and sexual abuse, depression and anxiety, alcohol and drug use, and other difficulties in a national sample of lesbian women. However, they did not examine the possible relationship between CSA and these other difficulties. Using the same sample, Hyman (2000) found that lesbian CSA experiencers reported more anxiety, depression, and suicidal ideation than nonexperiencers, as well as more health problems, less educational attainment, and lower annual earnings. Unfortunately, the range of emotional/behavioral sequelae to CSA examined in these studies was limited, and the number of adolescent women surveyed was relatively small.

There has also been surprisingly little research on the subjective experience of lesbian and bisexual females as it relates to CSA. In a qualitative study, Hall (1999) explored the sexual and relationship experiences of eight lesbian experiencers of CSA and found that almost all of the women interviewed experienced difficulties in their adult sexual relationships. These difficulties included: inability to acknowledge and express one's sexual needs, fear of initiating sexual encounters and replicating the abuse, difficulty differentiating sex, intimacy, and love, and a greater sense of normality, sexual freedom, and satisfaction within one's lesbian relationships (Hall, 1999). Although one might expect that CSA would affect a lesbian or bisexual young woman's sexual behavior, her feelings about her sexuality, or her "coming out" process, no published studies have examined the relationship between CSA and these other factors in larger samples or with quantitative analyses.

The current study sought to address these gaps in the literature by examining CSA in a national, nonclinical sample of lesbian and bisexual young women, ages 18-23, who were recruited over the Internet. We hypothesized that lesbian and bisexual females who were CSA experiencers would be more likely than nonexperiencers to report a range of emotional/behavioral difficulties. We also surmised that CSA would negatively impact a lesbian or bisexual young woman's sexuality development, and we therefore hypothesized that those participants who were experiencers would report that a CSA history had significantly affected their feelings about their sexuality or their "coming out" process.

METHODS

Recruitment

We posted an electronic mail message to LGB college organizations nationwide indicating that we were studying the possible effect of childhood and adolescent experiences on the well-being and "coming out" process of LGB individuals ages 18-23. (Several participants forwarded the message to acquaintances or friends, in effect creating a second wave of recruitment via "snowball sampling.") We specifically sampled this age range because we wanted participants to be as close to their childhood and adolescent experiences as possible, to minimize retrospective bias, while still being old enough to participate without parental consent.

Instrument

Participants volunteered to complete an online questionnaire which required approximately one hour of their time. The anonymous questionnaire contained quantitative and qualitative items about participant demographics, sexual orientation, sexual development, home environment, behavioral/emotional difficulties, victimization experiences, and social support. The questionnaire included both standardized instruments and measures created by the authors. As the study was designed to test a number of hypotheses not relevant to the current discussion, not all of the measures included in the questionnaire are described below.

As part of the questionnaire, we presented participants with a list of 19 problems culled from the LGB youth and trauma literatures and asked if they had experienced any of these difficulties during childhood or adolescence. (This measure was of our own design, as there are no standardized measures addressing all of these potential problem areas.) These experiences included: depression, anxiety, suicide attempt with no intent to die, suicide attempt with intent to die, self-injury, compulsive exercise, disordered eating, disturbance of body image, substance use problems, reckless driving, other risk-taking, school problems, unsafe sex, sexual behavior that led to pain or injury, having sex with strangers or other people who could be dangerous, being sexually active with multiple partners, dangerous activity, illegal activity, and running away. Participants were instructed to rate each of these experiences "at its worst" on a 7-point Likert scale from 1 ("not bad") to 7 ("very bad") or to indicate "N/A" if they had not had the experience during childhood or adolescence. For the purposes of this paper, participant ratings were re-coded as "yes" responses, and "N/A's" were re-coded as "no" responses.

To determine if they had a CSA history, we asked participants, "When you were a child or adolescent (below the age of 18), did someone(s) who was at least 5 years older than yourself or someone(s) whom you perceived as being more powerful ever encourage you or force you to have sexual contact with them?" We adapted this question from a prior study of CSA in gay and bisexual men (Bartholow et al., 1994). Of those participants who endorsed this question (CSA experiencers), we also asked, "Overall, do you feel that this sexual experience (or experiences) has affected your feelings about your sexuality or how you 'came out'?" and "If yes, how and why?" (For a complete description of the questionnaire, readers should contact the investigators.)

Procedures

In the recruitment message, we directed potential participants to the study URL address, where they could find information about the study, including information about the investigators, a description of the study and what participants could expect, consent-related information, and instructions for completing the questionnaire. Acknowledging that participation in such a study might bring up feelings and thoughts which could be distressing or uncomfortable, we also told potential participants that they could contact us for the names of helping professionals. In addition, we directed them to a listing of referral sources and hyperlinks for mental health, LGB, and trauma-related Websites. Potential participants needed to scroll through this information in order to access the questionnaire.

Although the data were not encrypted, we were nonetheless able to protect participant privacy because names and e-mail addresses did not get transmitted with their responses. Thus, we assured potential participants that their responses would be kept anonymous, provided that they did not include personal information that could identify them in their answers. We also reminded them that their participation was voluntary, and that they could choose not to answer specific questions or stop completing the survey at any time. Those individuals ages 18-23 who chose to participate thus provided implied consent if they completed all ten "pages" of the questionnaire and chose to submit their electronic responses.

When (and only if) all ten messages were received from a participant, we combined them, attached an identification number to that case, and entered the quantitative data into an SPSS file for analysis. We also separated the qualitative responses from the data files and coded them for common themes, with all authors being in agreement on the categorizations. We collected data from 4/5/99 through 6/22/99.

RESULTS

Participant Characteristics

We received complete data files from 433 individuals, 253 (58.4%) of whom were female. Of these young women, 15 (5.9%) indicated that they were questioning whether they were LGB and were thus omitted from subsequent analyses. In response to the CSA question, eleven (4.6%) of the remaining females indicated that they were "not sure" and were also omitted from the study. Thus, for the purposes of this paper, the final sample consisted of 227 young women, 86 (37.9%) of whom reported a CSA history.

The majority (80.2%) of study participants were white, with the remaining 45 (19.8%) females being persons of color or of mixed-race. The mean age of the sample was 20.30 years (SD = 1.73), with individuals well-distributed throughout the 18-23 age range. In terms of socioeconomic status (SES), 48 (21.1%) participants were from the lower and working classes, 102 (44.9%) were from the middle class, and 77 (33.9%) were from the upper-middle and upper classes. Thirty participants (13.2%) had completed 1-5 years of high school, 188 (82.8%) had completed 1-5 years of college, and 9 (4.0%) had completed some graduate school or had received a graduate degree. The median participant was a college sophomore. Our sample was national in scope, as participants represented 38 states from across the country and Washington, D.C. A majority (56.4%) of respondents described the community in which they lived as "urban," while 43.6% reported living in "rural" or "suburban" areas.

To determine if the CSA experiencers and young women without a CSA history ("nonexperiencers") were sufficiently similar, we ran a number of comparative statistics on the two groups. There were not significant differences between CSA experiencers and nonexperiencers with regards to race, age, SES, educational level, geographic region, or type of community (see Table 1). However, CSA experiencers did report being "out" to a higher percentage of people in their lives than nonexperiencers ($M_{CSA} = 57.56\%$, $SD_{CSA} = 27.86$; $M_{Non} = 48.87\%$; $SD_{Non} = 28.16$), $t(181.20) = 2.27$, $p \leq .05$). In addition, CSA experiencers reported feeling more comfortable being LGB than nonexperiencers, on a 7-point Likert scale from 1 ("extremely uncomfortable") to 7 ("extremely uncomfortable") ($M_{CSA} = 6.14$, $SD_{CSA} = .95$; $M_{Non} = 5.65$; $SD_{Non} = 1.19$), $t(225) = 3.27$, $p \leq .001$).

Emotional/Behavioral Difficulties

In support of our first hypothesis, chi-square analyses indicated that CSA experiencers ($n = 86$) were significantly more likely than nonexperiencers ($n = 141$) to report 13 of the 19 emotional/behavioral difficulties (see Table 2), with particularly strong associations between CSA and the four sexual risk-taking behaviors. Experiencers also reported significantly more total problems ($M_{CSA} = 9.13$, $SD_{CSA} = 4.35$; $M_{Non} = 6.39$, $SD_{Non} = 3.64$), $t(155.90) = 4.89$, $p \leq .0001$) and more total sexual risk-taking behaviors than their nonexperiencer

TABLE 1. Demographic Characteristics of Experiencers vs. Nonexperiencers

Demographic Variable	CSA Experiencers (n = 86)	Nonexperiencers (n = 141)
Race	White (77.9%) Person of color/mixed (22.1%)	White (81.6%) Person of color/mixed (18.4%)
Age	M = 20.41 (SD = 1.72)	M = 20.24 (SD = 1.74)
SES	Lower/working (23.3%) Middle (41.9%) Upper-middle/upper (34.9%)	Lower/working (19.9%) Middle (46.8%) Upper-middle/upper (33.3%)
Educational level	High school (14.0%) College (82.6%) Graduate (3.5%)	High school (12.8%) College (83.0%) Graduate (4.3%)
Geographic region	Northeast (29.8%) Middle states (11.9%) North central (25.0%) Northwest (7.1%) Southern (17.9%) Western (8.3%)	Northeast (27.8%) Middle states (11.3%) North central (20.3%) Northwest (19.5%) Southern (12.0%) Western (9.0%)
Community	Urban (51.8%) Rural or suburban (48.2%)	Urban (59.3%) Rural or suburban (40.7%)

counterparts (M_{CSA} = 1.63, SD_{CSA} = 1.43; M_{Non} = .77, SD_{Non} = 1.08), $t(143.77) = 4.81, p \leq .0001$).

CSA Impact on Feelings About Sexuality or "Coming Out" Process

Of those participants who reported a CSA history, we asked, "Overall, what effect has this sexual experience (or experiences) had on you?" on a 7-point Likert scale from 1 ("no effect") to 7 ("extremely negative"). The vast majority rated the experience as very negative ($M = 5.18$, $SD = 1.65$), with only 3 (3.6%) young women indicating that their experience had had "no effect" on them. In partial support of our second hypothesis, however, when asked whether they felt that a history of CSA had affected their feelings about their sexuality or how they "came out," only 39 (46.4%) of the experiencers indicated that it had.

What might differentiate those experiencers who felt that CSA had affected their feelings about their sexuality or "coming out" process from those who did not? Further quantitative analyses shed little light on this finding: although we expected that ratings of the overall effect of the CSA experience ($M_{Yes} = 5.46$, $SD_{Yes} = 1.43$; $M_{No} = 4.98$, $SD_{No} = 1.81$; $t(79) = 1.31$), total number of total emotional/behavioral problems reported ($M_{Yes} = 9.21$, $SD_{Yes} = 4.14$; M_{No} = 8.87, $SD_{No} = 4.55$; $t(82) = .35$), or total number of sexual risk-taking behaviors reported ($M_{Yes} = 1.67$, $SD_{Yes} = 1.46$; $M_{No} = 1.56$, $SD_{No} = 1.44$; $t(82) = .35$)

TABLE 2. Differences in Emotional/Behavioral Difficulties Between Experiencers and Nonexperiencers

Emotional/Behavioral Difficulties	% All	% CSA	% Non-CSA	X^2 (*df* = 1)
depression	94.7	94.2	95.0	n.s.
anxiety	81.9	88.4	78.0	3.87*
suicide attempt with no intent to die	48.5	57.0	43.3	4.02*
suicide attempt with intent to die	24.2	31.4	19.9	3.87*
self-injury	55.1	65.1	48.9	5.65*
compulsive exercise	21.1	30.2	15.6	6.86**
disordered eating	48.5	54.7	44.7	n.s.
body image disturbance	64.8	70.9	61.0	n.s.
substance use problems	33.0	45.3	25.5	9.48**
reckless driving	30.0	31.4	29.1	n.s.
other risk-taking	14.1	17.4	12.1	n.s.
school problems	26.0	32.6	22.0	n.s.
dangerous activity	32.2	44.2	24.8	9.18**
illegal activity	41.4	58.1	31.2	15.97****
running away	18.1	29.1	11.3	11.34***
unsafe sex	37.0	52.3	27.7	13.94****
sex–pain or injury	22.0	34.9	14.2	13.33****
sex–strangers or dangerous	20.3	31.4	13.5	10.62***
sex–multiple partners	30.0	44.2	21.3	13.36****

Note. * $p \leq .05$; ** $p \leq .01$; *** $p \leq .001$; **** $p \leq .0001$

might distinguish between the two groups, none of the group differences on these measures was statistically significant.

To understand better how and why some participants felt that CSA had affected their sexuality or "coming out" experience, we turned to a content analysis of the qualitative responses of those young women who had answered in the affirmative. We categorized their responses into several categories, based on common themes identified by the investigators (see Table 3). We did not consider these categories to be mutually exclusive (some of the lengthier responses fit into more than one) or exhaustive, but rather jumping-off points for further discussion and analysis. Not all participant responses were subject to categorization, as we selected only those themes that were touched upon by more than one participant.

TABLE 3. Qualitative Responses: How and Why CSA Affected Sexuality or "Coming Out" Experience

Theme	Example
Positive impact	The relationship in question . . . made me feel very positive about being queer.
Impact on timing or duration of experience	I understood what sex was at a very early age, and was therefore able to interpret my attraction for people of the same sex at an earlier age.
Sexual orientation as the/a reason for CSA	The first time I attempted to come out to someone . . . he sexually assaulted me.
Impact on relationships with men	It engendered a sense of distrust of the male sex drive and male sexuality on a whole.
Impact on sexuality but not sexual orientation	The childhood experiences have more to do with how I perceive my sexuality as a whole rather than its specific orientation.
Impact on sense of validity of own experience	It made me wonder if my feelings were invalid and whether I was/wasn't just afraid of men because of bad experiences.
Did CSA cause or affect sexual orientation?	I think that coming to terms with my abuse was a factor, although not the main one, behind my identifying as a lesbian.

A few participants reported that their experiences had affected their "coming out" process in a good way: "The relationship in question taught me a lot and helped me grow up a lot, and it also made me feel very positive about being queer. It gave me a chance to explore my sexual feelings"; "My first girlfriend when I was 17 was in her mid-twenties. It was a 'positive' experience." It is likely that these participants would not have self-identified as CSA experiencers. It would be useful to identify those potential factors (e.g., Female partner? Older age?) that led such young women to feel that their sexual experiences had positively impacted their sexuality or "coming out" process.

Some participants felt that CSA had contributed to earlier knowledge of their sexuality: "Unpleasant sex experiences forced me to think a lot about sex and what I thought about it . . . Since I already had to do work about sex, the LGB work was just another aspect"; "My indifference to sexual experiences with men made me consider my lesbian sexuality earlier and it made more sense"; "If anything, I understood what sex was at a very early age, and was therefore able to interpret my attraction for people of the same sex at an earlier age." Other young women felt that CSA had delayed or prolonged their "coming out" process: "Because this experience took away my power, both sexually and in terms of self-confidence, I became blind to anything about myself sexually other than pleasing men . . . and dismissed my sexual feelings for women as 'not real,' 'not legitimate,' and not anything to be believed in . . . it took me years to gain my power back"; "It made the coming out process a lot longer, as I did not want to fit the stereotype of being abused and becoming a lesbian." These responses made clear that CSA can affect the timing or length of some experiencers' "coming out" process in complicated ways.

A few participants reported that they were abused/assaulted because of their sexual minority identity: "I got raped many times because I acted too much like a boy and because I am a lesbian"; "The first time I attempted to come out to someone in high school, he sexually assaulted me–this made me much more careful and hesitant about coming out"; "I was raped by a man because I am a lesbian." These participants helped to highlight ways that identifying as lesbian or bisexual seems to place some young women at risk for sexual victimization or revictimization.

Many participants indicated that their CSA experiences had affected their relationship with men and to male sexuality: "I'm afraid of men"; "Makes it difficult to trust men"; "I have a huge fear of penetration"; "It engendered a sense of distrust of the male sex drive and male sexuality on a whole"; "Being raped has made me afraid to become physically intimate with men, so I often date women whom I can have a loving emotional relationship with along with a physical relationship"; "It resulted in a much greater sense of safety with women compared to men"; "I feel as though it has made me trust men much less than I actually should be able to." Thus, a number of our participants felt that CSA experiences had damaged their ability to trust men or to be involved romantically and sexually with men, perhaps irreparably so.

Some participants distinguished between sexuality and sexual orientation, reporting that CSA had affected their sexuality or sexual desire but not their sexual orientation: "I wouldn't say that this had any effect at all on my sexual orientation. As far as my sexuality as a whole is concerned, however, I could write an entire book about that"; "It has affected my feelings about and responses to sex in general, but it has not affected my coming out or my feelings about/responses to my (homo)sexuality"; "The childhood experiences have more to do with how I perceive my sexuality as a whole rather than its specific orientation"; "Although I do not think that it has affected my coming out process, I definitely think it instilled in me a feeling of sexual and physical inadequacy"; "The problem I have to deal with now is how that affected my sexuality . . . I'm so confused about my sexuality, NOT my sexual orientation, my sexuality." Several women thus felt that CSA had affected their experience of their sexual selves but not their choice of sexual partners.

Several young women bemoaned the fact that having experienced CSA influenced the responses of others and their own understanding of themselves: "One of my biggest fears, in fact, has been that people would think I am a lesbian simply because of the assaults–that my lesbianism is somehow less valid or 'pure' than someone without those experiences"; "It made me wonder if my feelings were invalid and whether I was/wasn't just afraid of men because of bad experiences"; "When people have doubts about whether or not I really am attracted to women when I come out to them, I can't really argue with them, because I have doubts myself. I wish I could know how I would feel if I weren't abused as a child–as I was meant to feel, without having been messed with." Thus, CSA led several participants to wrestle with feelings of invalidation–by themselves and by others–with regards to their sexuality.

Finally, several participants felt that a CSA history had contributed to their identification as lesbian or bisexual: "I don't think I buy the argument that I identify as a lesbian solely because I had so much sexual trauma in my childhood and adolescence, but of course it is related"; "At first I blamed my orientation on my abuse . . . but I know that I am mostly a lesbian"; "I think [molestation by a female] has some validity to why I feel an attraction to women, but I don't think it is the only reason I am attracted to females"; "I think that coming to terms with my abuse was a factor, although not the main one, behind my identifying as a lesbian." Other young women did not think that CSA had "caused" them to become lesbian or bisexual: "When I would tell people, they would sometimes say, 'Oh, that's probably why you're a lesbian' and I didn't think it was, and I still don't think that it is"; "I spent a lot of time justifying to myself that my lesbian sexuality hadn't been created or in any way influenced by [sexual abuse by an older male]. I don't believe his actions had any effect on my lesbianism"; "I am sure that regardless of that experience, I would have come to the realization that I love both men and women . . . I look back and I know that I have been attracted to women for as long as I can remember . . . and just the fact that I can still have feelings for men regardless of what those jerks did to me leaves me with no doubt that I DO really love men." Clearly, CSA forced many of the young women in our study to consider its potential impact on their lesbian or bisexual identification, and the range of subjective experiences reported demonstrates the lack of consensus on this issue.

DISCUSSION

Most LGB individuals are not childhood sexual abuse experiencers, and prior research has found no association between CSA and the development of an LGB sexual identity (Bell, Weinberg, & Hammersmith, 1981). Nonetheless, persistent myths remain in our society to suggest that LGB individuals are "made that way" by CSA experiences. Many researchers have not wanted to conduct studies which could be misinterpreted to contribute to this myth, and others have avoided exploring associations between CSA and sexual orientation due to the socially and politically sensitive nature of the topic. Our study examined the possible contribution of CSA to the difficulties and experience of some lesbian and bisexual young women. As hypothesized, we found a strong association between CSA and several emotional/behavioral problems reported for this population, suggesting that many of the difficulties found among these young women in the literature may be at least somewhat explained by trauma history. That we found particularly strong associations between CSA and sexual risk-taking is perhaps not surprising, since one might expect a linkage between CSA and subsequent sexual behavior. Nonetheless, this finding was especially significant, both because sexual activity is often a precursor to LGB identification, and because studies of high-risk sexual behavior in lesbian and bisexual young women are scarce (Anhalt & Morris, 1998). It is also important to note, however, that CSA was found to be a potential risk factor even for problems not as intuitively or theoretically linkable to sexual experiences (e.g., compulsive exercise, substance abuse, and running away).

In partial support of our second hypothesis, close to half of the experiencers in our sample indicated that CSA had affected their feelings about their sexuality or their "coming out" process. The qualitative data demonstrated that these young women understood the impact of CSA on their experience in rich and varied ways. This finding should remind us that quantitative statistics can blur important individual differences that have much to teach us about the complex relationship between CSA, sexuality, and the "coming out" process. That over half of the experiencers did not report that CSA had affected their feelings about their sexuality or their "coming out" process also suggests that we still have much to learn about factors which protect some experiencers from the potentially traumatic impact of CSA or which contribute to their resilience.

Limitations of the Study

Our study was an improvement over many prior studies of LGB youth. We limited gender and retrospective bias and we gathered data from a nonclinical sample. In addition, online data collection allowed us to reach a relatively large and geographically-diverse sample, to preserve anonymity, and to afford our participants greater freedom to respond honestly about sensitive topics. Nonetheless, our methodology secured a convenience sample which was predominately white, college-educated, Internet-savvy, and affiliated with LGB campus groups. Thus, the experiences of more marginalized young women (e.g., women of color) were not well represented, and these biases in our sample may have skewed the findings in some way. Importantly, we did not have a heterosexual comparison group against which to compare the rates of CSA and emotional/behavioral difficulties reported by our sample. Finally, the CSA experiencers in our sample were more "out" and more comfortable being LGB than their nonexperiencer counterparts, which may have influenced the study findings.

Our questionnaire could also have been improved; some sexual behavior classified either as "CSA" according to our definition or "risky" according to our survey items was not perceived as abusive or problematic by the participants, which may call into question some of our interpretations. (It could be argued, for example, that some forms of sexual risk-taking are a sign of healthy curiosity and sexual openness.) In addition, lack of information about the perpetrator (e.g., gender, relationship to participant) and about the type, number, frequency, severity, duration, and recency of abuse experiences also limited the hypotheses that could be tested and the conclusions that could be drawn. In particular, without knowing when the CSA experiences occurred, we could not definitively say whether CSA caused or contributed to participants' emotional/behavioral difficulties, or whether these problems put participants at greater risk for CSA. Further, unexamined third variables could arguably have placed some of the participants at risk for both victimization and later problems (Boney-McCoy & Finkelhor, 1996). Most of our qualitative analyses centered on responses to one open-ended item (the question of whether or not CSA had affected a young woman's experience of her sexuality or "coming out" process). As there was no opportunity for us to return to the participants for elaboration or clarification of their responses, the resulting analyses were necessarily preliminary. Finally, given the political and sensitive nature of the topic, the face validity of our questions about the impact of CSA on sexuality could have contributed to a response bias on the part of some participants.

Implications of Findings

Despite these limitations, our findings have important implications for prevention and intervention efforts with lesbian and bisexual young women. Certainly, internalized homophobia and experiences of LGB-related victimization and oppression contribute to the difficulties experienced by this population (Savin-Williams, 1994). However, these data suggest that therapists, outreach workers, and others must also be alert to the possibility of a CSA history when working with young lesbian and bisexual clients who have come to their attention due to emotional/behavioral problems. Indeed, we would recommend that young lesbian and bisexual clients be routinely screened for CSA, both because an undisclosed CSA history can place experiencers at risk for revictimization (Briere & Runtz, 1987), and because early identification might lower their risk for subsequent or more serious difficulties.

As noted by prior researchers (Finkelhor & Browne, 1985) and confirmed by some of our participants, sexual abuse can also contribute to confusion about sexual identity and sexual self-concept. In fact, a significant minority of our participants identified several important ways that CSA may affect a young woman's experience of her sexuality, including impacting the timing of her "coming out" process, damaging her relationships with men and male sexuality, impacting negatively her experience of her own sexuality, causing her and others to question the validity of her sexual experience, heightening her risk for (re-)victimization, and/or causing her to question whether or not CSA made her lesbian or bisexual. Thus, counselors working with lesbian and bisexual young women should consider exploring thoughts and feelings related to these themes with their clients. Importantly, therapists working with these clients must attend carefully to the subjective experience of each individual young woman, since the meanings that she attaches to her CSA experience (including positive ones) will undoubtedly determine some of its impact.

With regards to future research, we need to replicate and expand upon these findings with more methodologically-sound studies. It would be particularly interesting to compare rates of emotional/behavior difficulties in matched samples of LGB and heterosexual CSA experiencers and nonexperiencers. We also need to identify those moderating factors which would help to explain why some CSA experiencers did not report emotional/behavioral difficulties, and why so many experiencers reported no impact of CSA on their feelings about their sexuality or "coming out" process. It may be that some LGB experiencers do not recognize ways that CSA has affected their experience, or that some aspects of their experience are influenced by CSA while other aspects are not. It may also be that contrary to expectations of "traumatic sexualization" (Finkelhor & Browne, 1985), many lesbian and bisexual young women emerge from CSA experiences without their sexuality having been permanently or negatively affected. Hopefully, future studies of LGB CSA experiencers (including in-depth, qualitative interviews) will help us to identify those factors which mediate sexual abuse, behavior, desire, and orientation.

CONCLUSION

A thorough analysis of the impact of childhood sexual abuse has been neglected in prior studies of lesbian and bisexual young women. It is critical that childhood sexual abuse be considered in any examination or treatment of emotional/behavioral difficulties in this population, and in any attempts to devise sophisticated, nuanced models of lesbian and bisexual female sexuality development.

REFERENCES

Anhalt, K. & Morris, T.L. (1998). Developmental and adjustment issues of gay, lesbian, and bisexual adolescents: A review of the empirical literature. *Clinical Child and Family Psychology Review*, *1*, 215-230.

Bartholow, B.N., Doll, L.S., Joy, D., Douglas, J.M., Bolan, G., Harrison, J.S., Moss, P.M., & McKirnan, D. (1994). Emotional, behavioral, and HIV risks associated with sexual abuse among adult homosexual and bisexual men. *Child Abuse & Neglect*, *18*, 747-61.

Bell, A.P., Weinberg, M.S., & Hammersmith, S.K. (1981). *Sexual preference: Its development among men and women*. Bloomington, IN: Indiana University Press.

Boney-McCoy, S. & Finkelhor, D. (1996). Is youth victimization related to trauma symptoms and depression after controlling for prior symptoms and family relationships? A longitudinal, prospective study. *Journal of Consulting and Clinical Psychology*, *64*, 1406-1416.

Bradford, J., Ryan, C., & Rothblum, E.D. (1994). National lesbian health care survey: Implications for mental health care. *Journal of Consulting & Clinical Psychology*, *62*, 228-242.

Briere, J. & Runtz, M. (1987). Post sexual abuse trauma: Data and implications for clinical practice. *Journal of Interpersonal Violence*, *2*, 367-379.

Carballo-Dieguez, A. & Dolezal, C. (1995). Associations between history of childhood sexual abuse and adult HIV-risk sexual behavior in Puerto Rican men who have sex with men. *Child Abuse & Neglect*, *19*, 595-605.

Dempsey, C.L. (1994). Health and social issues of gay, lesbian, and bisexual adolescents. *Families in Society*, *75*, 160-167.

DiPlacido, J. (1998). Minority stress among lesbians, gay men, and bisexuals: A consequence of heterosexism, homophobia, and stigmatization. In G.M. Herek (Ed.), *Stigma and sexual orientation: Understanding prejudice against lesbians, gay men, and bisexuals*. Sage Publications: Thousand Oaks.

Finkelhor, D. & Browne, A. (1985). The traumatic impact of child sexual abuse: A conceptualization. *American Journal of Orthopsychiatry*, *55*, 530-541.

Gibson, P. (1989). Gay male and lesbian youth suicide. In M. Feinleib (Ed.), *Report of the Secretary's Task Force on Youth Suicide* (pp. 110-142). Washington: U.S. Department of Health and Human Services.

Hall, J. (1999). An exploration of the sexual and relationship experiences of lesbian survivors of childhood sexual abuse. *Sexual and Marital Therapy*, *14*, 61-70.

Hyman, B. (2000). The economic consequences of child sexual abuse for adult lesbian women. *Journal of Marriage and the Family*, *62*, 199-211.

Lenderking, W.R., Wold, C., Mayer, K.H., Goldstein, R., Losina, E., & Seage, G.R. (1997). Childhood sexual abuse among homosexual men: Prevalence and association with unsafe sex. *Journal of General Internal Medicine*, *12*, 250-253.

Lock, J. & Steiner, H. (1999). Gay, lesbian, and bisexual youth risks for emotional, physical, and social problems: Results from a community-based survey. *Journal of the American Academy of Child & Adolescent Psychiatry*, *38*, 297-304.

Neumann, D.A., Houskamp, B.M., Pollack, V.E., & Briere, J. (1996). The long-term sequelae of childhood sexual abuse in women: A meta-analytic review. *Child Maltreatment, 1*, 6-16.

Remafedi, G. (1987). Adolescent homosexuality: Psychosocial and medical implications. *Pediatrics, 79*, 331-337.

Remafedi, G., Farrow, J.A., & Deisher, R.W. (1993). Risk factors for attempted suicide in gay and bisexual youth. *Psychological perspectives on lesbian and gay male experiences* (pp. 486-499). New York: Columbia University Press.

Rotheram-Borus, M., Rosario, M., Meyer-Bahlburg, H., Koopman, C., Dopkins, S., & Davies, M. (1994). Sexual and substance use acts of gay and bisexual male adolescents in New York City. *Journal of Sex Research, 31*, 47-57.

Rotheram-Borus, M.J., Rosario, M., Van Rossem, R., Reid, H., & Gillis, R. (1995). Prevalence, course, and predictors of multiple problem behaviors among gay and bisexual male adolescents. *Developmental Psychology, 31*, 75-85.

Savin-Williams, R.C. (1994). Verbal and physical abuse as stressors in the lives of lesbian, gay male, and bisexual youths: Associations with school problems, running away, substance abuse, prostitution, and suicide. Special section: Mental health of lesbians and gay men. *Journal of Consulting and Clinical Psychology, 62*, 261-269.

Abuse, Social Support, and Depression Among HIV-Positive Heterosexual, Bisexual, and Lesbian Women

Nina A. Cooperman
Jane M. Simoni
David W. Lockhart

Nina A. Cooperman, PsyD, is currently a postdoctoral fellow in the Behavioral Sciences Training in Drug Abuse Research Program sponsored by the Medical and Health Research Association of New York City, Inc. She is also an adjunct instructor at the Robert Wood Johnson Medical School, University of Medicine and Dentistry.

Jane M. Simoni is Assistant Professor in the Department of Psychology at the University of Washington.

David W. Lockhart is a research consultant with the University of Washington Center for AIDS Research.

Address correspondence to: Jane M. Simoni, Assistant Professor, Department of Psychology, University of Washington, Box 351525, Seattle, WA 98105-1525 (E-mail: jsimoni@u.washington.edu).

This research was conducted in part while the first author was a Predoctoral and Postdoctoral Fellow in the Behavioral Sciences Training in Drug Abuse Research Program sponsored by the Medical and Health Research Association of New York City, Inc. and National Development and Research Institutes, Inc. with funding from the National Institute on Drug Abuse (5 T32 DA07233-09). Data collection was sponsored by an Aaron Diamond Postdoctoral Fellowship to the second author. Points of view and opinions in this paper do not necessarily represent the official positions of the United States Government, Medical and Health Research Association of New York City, Inc., and National Development Research Institutes, Inc.

[Haworth co-indexing entry note]: "Abuse, Social Support, and Depression Among HIV-Positive Heterosexual, Bisexual, and Lesbian Women." Cooperman, Nina A., Jane M. Simoni, and David W. Lockhart. Co-published simultaneously in *Journal of Lesbian Studies* (Harrington Park Press, an imprint of The Haworth Press, Inc.) Vol. 7, No. 4, 2003, pp. 49-66; and: *Trauma, Stress, and Resilience Among Sexual Minority Women: Rising Like the Phoenix* (ed: Kimberly F. Balsam) Harrington Park Press, an imprint of The Haworth Press, Inc., 2003, pp. 49-66. Single or multiple copies of this article are available for a fee from The Haworth Document Delivery Service [1-800-HAWORTH, 9:00 a.m. - 5:00 p.m. (EST). E-mail address: docdelivery@haworthpress.com].

http://www.haworthpress.com/store/product.asp?sku=J155

10.1300/J155v07n04_04

SUMMARY. A nonprobability sample of HIV-positive mostly African American and Puerto Rican women in New York City were surveyed regarding abusive experiences, social support, and depressive symptoms. Seventy-five percent reported experiencing physical or sexual abuse at some point in their lives. Multiple regression analyses controlling for relevant sociodemographic variables indicated that child physical and sexual abuse and adult sexual abuse were significantly associated with depressive symptomatology (i.e., CES-D scores). HIV-related social support had a significant negative correlation with CES-D scores but did not have a moderating impact on the effects of physical or sexual abuse. Lesbian/bisexual women reported higher rates of lifetime sexual and physical abuse than heterosexual women. However, there were no differences between the groups in total CES-D scores. Lesbian/bisexual women had significantly greater support from friends and groups/organizations than the heterosexual women. The implications of the findings for future research and the provision of services for HIV-positive women are considered.

KEYWORDS. Trauma, physical abuse, sexual abuse, social support, HIV/AIDS, psychosocial, depression, bisexual, lesbian, heterosexual, women of color, race/ethnicity

During the 1980s, women represented only 7% of those diagnosed with AIDS. By the year 2000, that percentage had quadrupled to 28%, and AIDS is now one of the leading causes of death among women 25-44 years of age in the United States (U.S.; Centers for Disease Control [CDC], 1999a; CDC, 2000). While African American and Hispanic women constitute less than 25% of the population of women in the U.S., they account for over 75% of AIDS cases among women. This group's relatively higher HIV risk has been attributed to such factors as poverty, drug use, poor healthcare, lack of education, and unemployment (Fernandez, 1995; Jemmott, Catan, Nyamathi, & Anastasia, 1995). Women living in impoverished African American or Hispanic communities have increased stressors and fewer resources compared to others, leaving them more vulnerable to HIV infection and less able to cope once infected.

Most HIV research and medical attention initially focused on those first infected with the virus–bisexual and gay men and male injection drug users

(Stevens, 1993). Furthermore, during the first decade of the HIV/AIDS epidemic, many women died from undiagnosed AIDS since AIDS-defining conditions did not include illnesses specific to women. It was not until 1993 that conditions specific to females (e.g., invasive cervical carcinoma and recurrent cervical dysplasia) were added (Morrow, 1995). Many women in the U.S., especially African American and Hispanic women, are living longer with HIV/AIDS. Researchers need to consider their unique qualities, stressors, strengths, and needs so that resources can be provided, life can be prolonged, and quality of life can be improved.

HIV Risk Among Lesbian and Bisexual Women

Given women's recent inclusion in the HIV/AIDS literature (Morrow, 1995) and the finding that heterosexual contact is the most frequent route of infection for women (CDC, 1999a), women who have sex with women (WSW) have been virtually ignored as a group at risk for contracting HIV. The CDC does not include female-to-female HIV transmission as an exposure category, and the prevalence of HIV infection among WSW is not specifically tracked. Even more problematically, since women are seldom asked about their partner's gender, WSW who report having partners who are injection drug users may be considered to be infected heterosexually.

While studies of female-to-female transmission of HIV are inconclusive (CDC, 1999b), several have shown that women who have sex with both women and men are more likely than women who have sex with only men to be HIV-positive and to engage in risky behavior such as drug use, prostitution, sex with multiple male partners, and unprotected sex (Gonzales, Washienka, Krone, Chapman, Arredondo, Huckeba, & Downer, 1999; Lemp, Jones, Kellogg, Nieri, Anderson, Withum, & Katz, 1995). Young, Friedman, Case, Asencio, and Clatts (2000) conducted a literature review that indicated high percentages of WSW among female injection drug users. The WSW were more likely than other women who use intravenous drugs to engage in risky injection behaviors and risky sexual behavior with men. They also reported higher percentages of HIV seroprevalence in WSW injection drug users than in injection drug users who do not report having sex with women.

Physical and Sexual Abuse and HIV Risk

Physical and sexual abuse has been associated with behaviors that can put an individual at risk for HIV infection, including injection drug use, lack of condom use, and multiple partners (Johnsen & Harlow, 1996; Thompson, Potter, Sanderson, & Maibach, 1997). Those who have been abused are more resistant to HIV education and prevention measures than those who have not been abused (Allers, Benjack, Rousey, & White, 1993). Miller (1999) explained that drug use is an easily accessible and immediate method of coping for female survivors of sexual abuse, and drug users with an abuse history are more likely to participate in needle sharing. While they may be aware of HIV, their drive to cope with psychological and emotional distress outweighs concerns about HIV risk. Miller also stated that abuse history has been linked to prostitution, and research has shown that sex workers are likely to participate in other risky behaviors such as inconsistent condom use and needle sharing. Physical and sexual abuse can impair self-esteem and interpersonal relating such that an abused individual will be less able to perceive risk in sexual relationships or to negotiate condom use and will be more likely to develop a pattern of revictimization (Johnsen & Harlow, 1996; Thompson et al., 1997).

Since those with an abuse history are more likely to engage in risky behavior, it is not surprising that women who have been physically or sexually abused constitute a large proportion of those infected with HIV. In fact, while percentages of child sexual abuse among women range from 7% to 36% (Finkelhor, 1994) and research suggests that between 20% and 33% of women will be physically abused by a partner during their lifetime (Cohen, Deamant, Barkan, Richardson, Young, Holman, Anastos, Cohn, & Melnick, 2000), studies of childhood sexual abuse prevalence among HIV-positive women indicate figures as high as 65% (Lodico & DiClemente, 1994). Cohen et al. (2000) found that among 1,288 HIV-positive women, 31% reported being sexually abused as a child and 66% reported a lifetime history of domestic violence. Liebschutz, Feinman, Sullivan, Stein, and Samet (2000) conducted chart reviews of 50 HIV-positive women and found evidence of sexual or physical abuse in 68% of the sample. However, only 46% reported an abuse history during an interview, indicating that patients are likely to underreport abuse experiences to researchers and actual levels may be even higher than studies suggest.

Abuse, Depression, and Social Support Among HIV-Positive Women

Sexual abuse is related to higher levels of depression among clinical and nonclinical samples (Finkelhor & Browne, 1986). Research indicates that stressful life experiences are associated with greater psychological distress among those with HIV (Patterson, Semple, Temoshok, Atkinson, McCutchan, Straits-Troster, Chandler, & Grant, 1993). Consequently, physical and sexual abuse is likely to be associated with higher levels of depressive symptomatology among HIV-positive women. Moreover, depression could be associated with suicidal ideation that leads to self-destructive HIV-risk behavior (e.g., sharing needles, trading sex for drugs; Miller [1999]). If a woman does not value life or if the immediate alleviation of negative feelings is primary, she will be less likely to consider HIV prevention behaviors.

Given the levels of depression among those with an abuse history and their tendency for risky behavior and self-destruction, understanding the prevalence of abuse and its relationship to depression among those who are HIV-positive is important to inform interventions that can aid well-being and prevent further spread of the disease. Furthermore, depressive symptomatology associated with an abuse history could have implications for medication adherence and resulting physical health in the HIV-positive population (Catz, Kelly, Bogart, Benotsch, & McAuliffe, 2000).

Psychosocial resources such as social support can provide protection from the negative outcomes associated with stressful life events such as physical and sexual abuse (Peterson, Folkman, & Bakeman, 1996). Cohen and Wills (1985) proposed that social support can have an impact on well-being through direct beneficial effects or through a buffering of the impact of stressful experiences. Among the HIV-positive population, research has shown that social support buffers the depression, physical complaints, and disease progression that are associated with life stress. For example, Leserman, Jackson, Petitto, Golden, Silva, Perkins, Cai, Folds, and Evans (1999) found that among HIV-positive men, cumulative lifetime stressful experiences, greater depressive symptomatology, and decreased social support were all associated with an advancement of HIV to AIDS. Another study found that lower satisfaction with social support and higher cumulative life stress were related to an acceleration of HIV to AIDS (Leserman, Petitto, Golden, Gaynes, Gu, Perkins, Silva, Folds, & Evans, 2000).

Abuse, Depression, and Social Support Among Lesbian and Bisexual Women

Since studies have shown that WSW exhibit higher levels of HIV risk behaviors that are also associated with abuse, further investigation of abuse experiences and sexual orientation could provide information that would be valuable for HIV prevention and treatment services. Research regarding the relationship between abuse history and sexual orientation has been contradictory and inconclusive. Some researchers have found higher percentages of physical and sexual abuse among lesbians than among heterosexual women (D'Augelli, 1996; Duncan, 1990; Roberts & Sorensen, 1999); other researchers have not found a relationship between abuse history and sexual orientation (Brannock & Chapman, 1990). The National Lesbian Health Care Survey, a community survey of 1,925 lesbians, found that 37% reported a lifetime history of physical abuse, 19% experienced incest, and 32% had been sexually attacked or raped as a child or adult (Bradford, Ryan, & Rothblum, 1997).

Gundlach (1977) conducted a study of 233 heterosexual and 225 lesbian women and found that an equal proportion of the lesbian and heterosexual women had experienced rape. Of the women who had been sexually assaulted by a stranger as a child, 50% were heterosexual and 50% were lesbian. However, of the 17 women who experienced childhood sexual abuse by a relative or close family friend, all but one identified as lesbian. Tjaden, Thoennes, and Allison (1999) found that based on information from the National Violence Against Women Survey, individuals who lived with a same-sex intimate partner were more likely to have been raped or physically assaulted as a child and as an adult than those who were married or cohabitating with an opposite-sex partner.

Research has suggested that social stress may be related to increases in psychological distress and that the stigma associated with a lesbian or bisexual identity may lead to increases in depression and anxiety (Cochran, 2001). Based on a review of several population-based studies, Cochran (2001) reported a greater lifetime risk of major depression and other psychiatric disorders among lesbians and gay men than among heterosexuals. The National Lesbian Health Care Survey indicated that one-third of the respondents had experienced a long period of depression or sadness (Bradford, Ryan, & Rothblum, 1997). However, given the broad definition of depression in the study, the percentages were not dissimilar to those reported by heterosexual women.

Social support negatively correlated with depression in a sample of lesbian women (Ayala & Coleman, 2000). Women who were in a relationship were less likely to be depressed, and social support from friends and family was negatively correlated with depression. However, according to the authors, lesbians may have more difficulty obtaining social support from family due to heterosexism and may turn to friends or gay and lesbian communities to develop "alternative families." Bradford, Ryan, and Rothblum (1997) found lesbians to have a variety of social supports and connections, but most of their support came from within the lesbian community and not from family members or coworkers.

HIV-positive lesbian and bisexual women of color not only have to deal with finding a voice in the majority culture and the HIV-positive community, they also must struggle for acceptance and acknowledgement in their own ethnic communities (Gonzalez & Espin, 1996; Jones & Hill, 1996). Research that focuses on the unique stressors and coping of HIV-positive lesbian and bisexual women of color is virtually nonexistent. The purpose of the present study was to fill this gap by acknowledging and describing some of the issues and strengths of a group of HIV-positive women, many of whom are dealing with double, triple, or quadruple minority status.

In the current study, we focused on the physical and sexual abuse histories, social support, and depression levels among 373 HIV-positive women of color. This information was part of a larger data set assessing sexual behaviors, well-being, and coping among HIV-positive women. In line with previous research, we hypothesized high frequencies of abuse, direct associations between abuse and depression, and both a general protective and stress-buffering effect of social support. Finally, with the purpose of providing further data on differences in abuse, mental health, and social resources between heterosexual and lesbian/bisexual women, we divided the sample based on sexual orientation and looked for differences in these variables.

METHODS

Procedures

Participants were recruited at outpatient HIV clinics, community-based AIDS organizations, and scatter-site housing in the New York metropolitan area. Fliers were posted and participants were notified about the study through word-of-mouth. In order to be eligible for the study, participants needed to be at least 18 years of age, have been diagnosed with HIV at least three months prior to participation, be able to give informed consent, and speak either English or Spanish. Interviews were conducted face-to-face by trained interviewers that included women from the HIV-positive community (Simoni, Weinberg, & Nero, 1999). The purpose, risks, and benefits of the study were described to each participant and informed consent was obtained. Most of the interviews were conducted on-site. Participants had a choice of whether to be interviewed in English or Spanish and were given $10, 2 tokens for public transportation, an AIDS information booklet, and a list of low-cost referrals to mental health and social service agencies and resources for their participation.

Participants

The sample of 373 women included 41% who were HIV-positive and asymptomatic, 35% who were HIV-positive and symptomatic, and 25% with an AIDS diagnosis. Self-identified risks for HIV transmission were unprotected sex with an intravenous drug user (48%), unprotected sex with a non-intravenous drug user (36%), intravenous drug use (36%), and blood transfusions (8%; note that participants could check all that applied). Participants were non-Hispanic African American (44%), Hispanic (mostly Puerto Rican; 25%), both Hispanic and African American (17%), non-Hispanic Caucasian (8%), American Indian

(2%), Asian (.3%), or some other race/ethnicity (4%). Age ranged from 18 to 66 years, with a mean of 39.6. Participants had an average of 11.2 years of education. Approximately 12% had less than a high school education, 50% had a high school diploma or GED as their highest level of education, 11% had some college or a bachelor's degree, and 2% had earned a graduate degree. Seventy-nine percent were unemployed, and 47% had a household monthly income of less than $500.

Over half of the participants (52%) were never legally married, 12% were legally married, and 36% were currently separated, divorced, or widowed. Among the 54% who reported having a steady partner, 84% reported having a male partner, 14% reported having a female partner, and 2% reported having both a male and female partner. In terms of sexual orientation, 74% considered themselves to be only heterosexual. The remaining women considered themselves to be more heterosexual than homosexual (9%), equally heterosexual and homosexual (6%), more homosexual than heterosexual (3%), or only homosexual (8%).

Measures

Abuse history. We assessed the frequency of physical and sexual abuse in childhood (i.e., before the age of 16 years) and adulthood (i.e., since the age of 16 years) with four items rated from 1 (*never*) to 7 (*> 20 times*). Specifically, we asked, "How many times have you been physically hurt, attacked, or abused or had your life threatened by anyone (including a family member or stranger) before you were 16 years old?" and "How many times were you sexually abused or raped by anyone (including a family member or stranger) before you were 16 years old?" Similar questions were asked about physical and sexual abuse since the age of 16.

Depressive symptomatology. Depression was measured with the Center for Epidemiologic Studies Depression Scale (CES-D; Radloff, 1977). This scale measures depressive symptomatology during the last week on a scale from 0 (*rarely or none of the time, less than one day in the past week*) to 3 (*most or all of the time, 5-7 days in the past week*). The measure consists of 20 questions with a potential for a minimum score of 0 and a maximum score of 60. Studies have supported the internal consistency, construct validity, and reliability of the CES-D (Radloff, 1977). In our sample, Cronbach's alpha was .83.

Social support. The UCLA Social Support Inventory was used to measure social support. The inventory asks about various types of HIV-related social support (i.e., information and advice, tangible assistance, encouragement and reassurance) provided by (a) friends, (b) relatives, (c) partners, and (d) groups or organizations during the past 30 days. Participants rated support received from 1 (*never*) to 5 (*very often*). Studies have supported the internal consistency, construct validity, and reliability of the UCLA Social Support Inventory (Schwarzer, Dunkel-Schetter, & Kemeny, 1994). In our sample, Cronbach's alphas were: .88 (friends), .90 (relatives), .92 (groups or organizations), and .96 (partners).

Sexual orientation. Sexual orientation was measured with a modified item from Kinsey, Pomeroy, and Martin (1948) that rated sexual orientation on a continuum from 1 (*only heterosexual*) to 5 (*only homosexual*). Since those who identified as *mainly heterosexual, equally heterosexual and homosexual, mainly homosexual, and only homosexual* had similarly high rates of sexual and physical abuse as compared to those who identified as *only heterosexual*, a dichotomous variable was created that indicated whether subjects were 0 (*only heterosexual*) or 1 (*lesbian/bisexual*).

RESULTS

Abuse, Depression, and Social Support: Descriptive Statistics

As hypothesized, abuse was highly prevalent in this sample: 75% reported physical or sexual abuse during their lifetime. With respect to child abuse, 46% percent had been physically abused and 42% sexually abused. In adulthood, 60% had been physically abused and 45% sexually abused. An ANOVA indicated that there were no significant differences in abuse based on race or ethnic background. On average, total depression scores within the sample were high ($M = 21.36$, $SD = 12.94$; range 0 to 56) with 61% of the study participants surpassing the traditional cutoff (16) for clinical depression (Radloff, 1977). The mean levels of HIV-related social support varied by source: groups or organizations ($M = 3.24$, $SD = 1.32$); followed by partners ($M = 2.75$, $SD = 1.61$) and friends ($M = 2.75$, $SD = 1.19$); and relatives ($M = 2.63$, $SD = 1.32$). Paired t tests showed that the only significant difference was between social support from groups/organizations and relatives ($t = -7.24$, $p < .001$).

Physical and Sexual Abuse Predicting Depression

We first explored possible associations between the sociodemographic indicators (i.e., race/ethnicity, age, education, work status, relationship status, and disease status) and the main variables of abuse and depression. Bivariate correlations and ANOVAS indicated only two significant findings: those who had higher education ($r = -.12$, $p < .05$) or were employed ($F = 2.51$, $p < .05$) were less depressed.

A series of five separate linear regression analyses were then conducted to determine whether different types of abuse predicted depression in this sample. Education and work status were entered as covariates. Child physical abuse ($\beta = .213, p < .001$); child sexual abuse ($\beta = .170, p < .001$); adult sexual abuse ($\beta = .127, p < .05$); and any sexual or physical abuse ($\beta = .178, p < .001$) had small but significant correlations with depression. Adult physical abuse was not significantly associated with depression ($\beta = .056, p = .29$). R^2 ranged from .039 for adult physical abuse to .076 for child physical abuse.

Protective and Buffering Effects of Social Support

A Pearson correlation revealed that total HIV-related social support was negatively associated with depression ($r = -.168, p < .01$), suggesting a protective or main effect of social support on depression.

We next assessed a possible buffering effect of social support. In other words, we wanted to determine whether the association between abuse and depression was greater among those with less support relative to those with more support. Therefore, we ran two linear regression models–one including the main effect of abuse and the main effect of social support with depression as the dependent variable and the other including both main effects as well as their interaction, again with depression as the dependent variable.

Clear evidence of a buffering effect from these analyses would consist of a significant coefficient for the interaction of abuse and social support on depression in the interaction regression model. Our results indicated that the interaction term was nonsignificant. However, the confidence interval for the interaction term was (−0.297, 0.032), which is wide and includes values that are large relative to the overall effect of abuse on depression in the main effects regression model. This can be interpreted to mean that among those with the most social support, the effect of abuse on depression is about one-third less than among those with the least social support. These findings indicate our lack of power to detect a buffering effect.

Therefore, we can conclude that social support has a protective or main effect on depression in our sample, but it is not clear whether this arises from a general protective effect, a buffering effect, or a combination of the two.

Sexual Orientation Group Differences

Sociodemographics (i.e., race/ethnicity, age, education, work status, relationship status, disease status); physical and sexual abuse history; social support; and depression were compared among women who identified as only heterosexual (n = 274) and women who identified as lesbian/bisexual (i.e., mainly heterosexual, equally heterosexual and homosexual, mainly homosexual, or only homosexual; n = 95). Chi-squares, t tests and ANOVAs indicated that no sociodemographic differences were significant. Therefore, none were included in future analyses of sexual orientation.

As shown in Table 1, levels of abuse were consistently higher among lesbian/bisexual women than heterosexual women. Note that fully 94% of the lesbian/bisexual women reported an abuse history. Table 2 displays results of a MANOVA indicating that the lesbian/bisexual group had significantly higher frequencies of all types of abuse. A *t* test (Table 2) indicated that no significant differences existed between the heterosexual women and the lesbian/bisexual women in terms of depression. Finally, a MANOVA with the social support variables indicated that, compared to heterosexual women, lesbian/bisexual women reported significantly higher levels of social support from friends and from groups/organizations in the past 30 days.

DISCUSSION

This study examined the relationships among physical and sexual abuse, social support, and depression within a sample of 373 HIV-positive mostly African American and Puerto Rican women from New York City. Differences based on sexual orientation were explored. The results indicated high levels of both physical and sexual abuse that are consistent with, and in some cases even higher, than those in other published studies with HIV-positive or ethnic minority samples (Bedimo, Kissinger, & Bessinger, 1997; Cohen et al., 2000; Liebschutz et al., 2000; Hien & Bukszpan, 1999). While this study had a mostly ethnic minority sample, research suggests that factors other than race/ethnicity are contributing to the increase in abuse. In a study comparing HIV-positive to HIV-negative women, Wyatt et al. (2002) found that abuse predicted HIV-risk behavior independently of race, and HIV-positive women

TABLE 1. Physical and Sexual Abuse Prevalence by Sexual Orientation

	Sexual Orientation			
Type of abuse	Heterosexual (n = 274)		Lesbian/Bisexual (n = 95)	
	%	*n*	%	*n*
Child physical abuse	42	116	56	53
Child sexual abuse	38	103	55	52
Adult physical abuse	55	150	75	71
Adult sexual abuse	39	106	65	62
Any physical or sexual abuse	69	188	94	89

TABLE 2. Differences in Abuse, Social Support, and Depression by Sexual Orientation

	Heterosexual (n = 274)		Lesbian/Bisexual (n = 95)		Between Groups
	M	*SD*	*M*	*SD*	*F*
Frequency of Abuse[a]					7.46[b]***
Child sexual abuse	1.97	1.63	2.51	1.92	6.84**
Child physical abuse	2.35	1.96	3.09	2.30	8.93**
Adult physical abuse	2.67	1.92	3.68	2.13	18.16***
Adult sexual abuse	1.85	1.33	2.76	1.88	25.74***
Frequency of Social Support[c]					2.49[d]*
Social support from friends	2.65	1.20	3.03	1.16	6.72**
Social support from relatives	2.60	1.35	2.70	1.29	.40
Social support from partners	2.66	1.60	2.99	1.62	2.48
Social support from groups/organizations	3.14	1.35	3.51	1.23	5.25*
					t
Depression[e]	21.54	12.53	20.96	14.25	.35

[a] Abuse scores range from 1 (*never*) to 7 (*> than 20 times*).
[b] Multivariate *F*, including all abuse variables.
[c] Social support scores range from 1 (*never*) to 5 (*very often*) during past 30 days.
[d] Multivariate *F*, including all social support variables.
[e] Total CES-D scores range from 0 to 60.
*$p < .05$; **$p < .01$; ***$p < .001$.

had more severe histories of abuse than HIV-negative women, regardless of ethnicity.

The hypothesis that abuse would be associated with depression was mostly supported, with the exception of adult physical abuse. A possible reason for this finding may be the broad wording of the question about physical abuse. The severity of physical harm or threat and one's relationship with the perpetrator could differentially impact physical and psychological health. Also, while those who were abused as a child are often vulnerable to repeated abuse as an adult, some members of this sample may have been physically assaulted first and only as an adult. Research indicates that a single physical assault that occurs during adulthood has less of an impact than childhood or repeated abuse. In a study of 633 women, Messman-Moore, Long, and Siegfried (2000) found that the women who had been abused as a child and retraumatized as an adult were more likely to be depressed than those who only experienced abuse during adulthood. In fact, the women who reported only adult assault were no more likely to be distressed than the women who were never abused.

In support of previous research (Cohen & Wills, 1985; Peterson, Folkman, & Bakeman, 1996), HIV-related social support had a significant negative relationship with depression in this sample. However, unlike in other studies that have shown a buffering relationship between stress and depression (Patterson et al., 1993), it is unclear whether HIV-related social support served as a buffer between abuse and depression. According to Cohen and Wills (1985), this may be due to the fact that the social support being measured in this sample is HIV-related and not specific to physical or sexual abuse. Their model states that a buffering effect will only be shown when the moderator is specific and matched to the stressor. Also, our study lacked power to determine the precise nature of the relationship between support and depression.

Significantly higher frequencies of abuse were found among those who identified as bisexual or lesbian as compared to heterosexual. In fact, the prevalence of physical or sexual abuse among the bisexual and lesbian women in this sample was also higher than among lesbian women in the general population (Bradford, Ryan, & Rothblum, 1997). The National Lesbian Health Care Survey found that African American and Latina lesbian women had significantly higher rates of abuse than White, lesbian women (Bradford, Ryan, & Rothblum, 1997). However, since the sample in this study consisted of mostly minority women, it is unlikely that the increased prevalence of sexual and physical abuse among the lesbian/bisexual women is related to ethnic or racial differences. Moreover, the direct association between race/ethnicity on abuse was nonsignificant.

Theorists have offered some explanations about the connection between physical and sexual abuse and sexual orientation. Due to discrimination and homophobia, being a sexual minority may leave one vulnerable to attack (D'Augelli, 1996). Others posited a different temporal association between awareness of one's sexual orientation and the experience of abuse. Specifically, Finkelhor (1984) has suggested that women who have been abused by men during their childhood will conclude that men are undesirable and choose women as sexual partners. According to Herman (1981), choosing to avoid men is an adaptive response to a traumatic experience. Courtois (1988) suggested that sexual abuse is related to promiscuity, and that some women may be "indiscriminant in choosing the sex of the partner just as they are in choosing partners in general" (p. 108). Maltz (1987) speculated that there are subgroups of lesbian and bisexual abuse survivors. "The first group of women are lesbians who also happen to be incest survivors. They would have been lesbian with or without the incest experience. The other group of women may be basically heterosexual or bisexual and have been open to experimentation with female partners as part of their healing process" (p. 72). Maltz believes that early incest experiences may confuse sexual orientation development for both heterosexual and lesbian women, blocking from awareness the heterosexuals' preference for men and the lesbians' preference for women.

In sum, the literature regarding the relationship between abuse history and sexual orientation is inconclusive and one needs to be careful about making causal attributions or inferring that lesbian or bisexual identity is a response to a pathological circumstance. While the results of this study indicate relationships between abuse history and sexual orientation, they are limited to the HIV-positive population. Further research is necessary to better understand sexual orientation and its connection to abuse experiences.

Interestingly, while abuse was related to increased depression and the lesbian/bisexual women were more likely than the heterosexual women to report abuse, there were no differences between the groups in terms of depression. This may be due to the relatively high levels of depression and symptomatology that exist in the overall sample. All members of the sample are HIV-positive and many are struggling with depression, including those without an abuse history. Therefore, lesbian/bisexual women may experience more depression because of their abuse but this increase is not significantly greater. An alternative explanation relates to the higher levels of social support reported by the lesbian/bisexual women than by the heterosexual women. While the lesbian/bisexual women did not have significantly greater social support from relatives or partners, they did have significantly more social support from friends and groups/organizations than the heterosexual women. It is possible that the women who identified as lesbian/bisexual actively participated in the gay, lesbian, and bisexual communities and thereby received greater HIV-related support. Social support was negatively correlated with depression in this sample and the increased HIV-related social support from friends and groups/organizations among the lesbian/bisexual women could have prevented an increase in depression, despite greater levels of abuse.

This study has several limitations. First, participants were recruited through purposive and convenience sampling and, therefore, the results cannot be generalized to all HIV-positive women. Second, the measure of social support was limited to HIV-related social support; perhaps a broader measure could have better tapped into the role of social support in psychological adaptation. Third, when comparing the groups based on self-identified sexual orientation, the lesbian and bisexual women were grouped together. Research has indicated that there may be differences between these groups of women (Fox, 1996). Finally, our method of assessing physical and sexual abuse may have had an impact on the results for several reasons: (a) the reports of abuse were retrospective, which could have decreased accuracy; (b) participants did not know the interviewers and this may have affected their willingness to divulge sensitive and emotionally charged information; (c) the items assessing sexual and physical abuse were rather broad and may have been interpreted in varying ways by participants; and (d) these items were single-item measures and not from a standardized scale with known reliability and validity.

Despite these limitations, the results provide information that can assist with the development of intervention strategies. Given the prevalence of physical and sexual abuse among HIV-positive women, women who have an abuse history should be targeted for HIV education and prevention measures. However, research indicates that they are more likely to be resistant to HIV prevention messages due to the impulsivity and immediate need to alleviate negative feelings that is associated with abuse (Allers et al., 1993). Therefore, the abuse history, consequences, and resistance should be addressed and treated in combination with the implementation of HIV prevention interventions. Many women living with HIV/AIDS have an abuse history. Providers need to assess abuse when working with HIV-positive women, since it could have an impact on physical and psychological health (Simoni & Ng, 2002). Therapy that focuses on abuse experiences among HIV-positive women has the potential to enhance well-being, encourage medication compliance, and encourage adaptive coping behaviors to lower the risk of transmission. This study suggests that social support could be one avenue for such intervention, with support groups that focus on abuse a potentially helpful strategy. Also, since lesbian/bisexual women may have higher levels of sexual and physical abuse, they are more likely to be suffering from its psychological and physical consequences and to be participating in risky behavior. They should be targeted for prevention and intervention. Support networks that address the specific needs of lesbian and bisexual women would be beneficial and could form part of the psychological and medical response that this research suggests these women deserve.

REFERENCES

Allers, C., Benjack, K., White, J., & Rousey, J. (1993). HIV vulnerability and the adult survivor of childhood sexual abuse. *Child Abuse and Neglect, 17*, 291-298.

Ayala, J. & Coleman, H. (2000). Predictors of depression among lesbian women. *Journal of Lesbian Studies, 4(3)*, 71-86.

Bedimo, A., Kissinger, P., & Bessinger, R. (1997). History of sexual abuse among HIV-infected women. *International Journal of STD & AIDS, 8*, 332-335.

Bradford, J., Ryan, C., & Rothblum (1997). National lesbian health care survey: Implications for mental health care. *Journal of Lesbian Studies, 1(2)*, 217-249.

Brannock, J. & Chapman, B. (1990). Negative sexual experiences with men among heterosexual women and lesbians. *Journal of Homosexuality, 19(1)*, 105-110.

Catz, S., Kelly, J., Bogart, L., Benotsch, E., & McAuliffe, T. (2000). Patterns, correlates, and barriers to medication adherence among persons prescribed new treatments and HIV disease. *Health Psychology, 19(2)*, 124-133.

Centers for Disease Control and Prevention (1999a). *HIV/AIDS among U.S. women: Minority and young women at continuing risk.*

Centers for Disease Control and Prevention (1999b). *HIV/AIDS and U.S. women who have sex with women (WSW).*

Centers for Disease Control and Prevention (2000). *HIV/AIDS surveillance report, midyear edition, 12(1).*

Cochran, S. (2001). Emerging issues in research on lesbians' and gay men's mental health: Does sexual orientation really matter? *American Psychologist, 56(11)*, 929-947.

Cohen, M., Deamant, C., Barkan, S., Richardson, J., Young, M., Holman, S., Anastos, K., Cohn, J., & Melnick, S. (2000). Domestic violence and childhood sexual abuse in HIV-infected women and women at risk for HIV. *American Journal of Public Health, 90(4)*, 560-565.

Cohen, S. & Wills, T. (1985). Stress, social support, and the buffering hypothesis. *Psychological Bulletin, 98(2)*, 310-357.

Courtois, C. (1988). *Healing the incest wound: Adult survivors in therapy*. New York: W.W. Norton.

D'Augelli, A. (1996). Lesbian, gay, and bisexual development during adolescence and young adulthood. In R. Cabaj & T. Stein (Eds.), *Textbook of homosexuality and mental health* (pp. 267-288). Washington, DC: American Psychiatric Press.

Duncan, D. (1990). Prevalence of sexual assault victimization among heterosexual and gay/lesbian university students. *Psychological Reports, 66*, 65-66.

Fernandez, M. (1995). Latinas and AIDS, challenges to HIV prevention efforts. In A. O'Leary & L. Jemmott (Eds.), *Women at risk, issues in the primary prevention of AIDS* (pp. 159-174). New York and London: Plenum Press.

Finkelhor, D. (1984). *Child sexual abuse, new theory and research.* New York: The Free Press.

Finkelhor, D. (1994). The international epidemiology of child sexual abuse. *Child Abuse & Neglect, 18(5)*, 409-417.

Finkelhor, D. & Browne, A. (1986). Impact of child sexual abuse: A review of the research. *Psychological Bulletin, 99(1)*, 66-77.

Fox, R. (1996). Bisexuality, an examination of theory and research. In R. Cabaj & T. Stein (Eds.), *Textbook of homosexuality and mental health* (pp. 147-163). Washington, DC: American Psychiatric Press.

Gonzales, V., Washienka, K., Krone, M., Chapman, L., Arredondo, E., Huckeba, H., & Downer, A. (1999). Sexual and drug-use risk factors for HIV and STDs: A comparison of women with and without bisexual experiences. *American Journal of Public Health, 89(12)*, 1841-1846.

Gonzalez, F. & Espin, O. (1996). Latino men, Latina women, and homosexuality. In R. Cabaj & T. Stein (Eds.), *Textbook of homosexuality and mental health* (pp. 583-601). Washington, DC: American Psychiatric Press.

Gundlach, R. (1977). Sexual molestation and rape reported by homosexual and heterosexual women. *Journal of Homosexuality, 2(4)*, 367-384.

Herman, J. (1981). *Father-daughter incest*. Cambridge, MA: Harvard University.

Hien, D. & Bukszpan, C. (1999). Interpersonal violence in a "normal" low-income control group. *Women & Health, 29(4)*, 1-16.

Jemmott, L., Catan, V., Nyamathi, A., & Anastasia, J. (1995). African American women and risk of sexually transmitted HIV infection. In A. O'Leary & L. Jemmott (Eds.), *Women at risk, issues in the primary prevention of AIDS* (pp. 159-174). New York and London: Plenum Press.

Johnsen, L. & Harlow, L. (1996). Childhood sexual abuse linked with adult substance use, victimization, and aids-risk. *AIDS Education and Prevention, 8(1)*, 44-57.

Jones, B. & Hill, M. (1996). African American lesbians, gay men, and bisexuals. In R. Cabaj & T. Stein (Eds.), *Textbook of homosexuality and mental health* (pp. 549-561). Washington, DC: American Psychiatric Press.

Kinsey, A., Pomeroy, W., & Martin, C. (1948). *Sexual behavior in the human male*. Philadelphia: Saunders.

Lemp, G., Jones, M., Kellogg, T., Nieri, G., Anderson, L., Withum, D., & Katz, M. (1995). HIV seroprevalence and risk behaviors among lesbians and bisexual women in San Francisco and Berkeley, California. *American Journal of Public Health, 85(11)*, 1549-1552.

Leserman, J., Jackson, E., Petitto, J., Golden, R., Silva, G., Perkins, D., Cai, J., Folds, J., & Evans, D. (1999). Progression to AIDS: The effects of stress, depressive symptoms, and social support. *Psychosomatic Medicine, 61*, 397-406.

Leserman, J., Petitto, J., Golden, R., Gaynes, B., Gu, H., Perkins, D., Silva, S., Folds, J., & Evans, D. (2000). Impact of stressful life events, depression, social support, coping, and cortisol on progression to AIDS. *American Journal of Psychiatry, 157(8)*, 1221-1228.

Liebschutz, J., Feinman, G., Sullivan, L., Stein, M., & Samet, J. (2000). Physical and sexual abuse in women infected with the human immunodeficiency virus, increased illness and health care utilization. *Archives of Internal Medicine, 160*, 1659-1664.

Lodico, M. & DiClemente, R. (1994). The association between childhood sexual abuse and prevalence of HIV-related risk behaviors. *Clinical Pediatrics, 33(8)*, 498-502.

Maltz, W. (1987). *Incest and sexuality: A guide to understanding and healing*. Lexington, MA: Lexington Books.

Messman-Moore, T., Long, P., & Siegfried, N. (2000). The revictimization of child sexual abuse survivors: An examination of the adjustment of college women with child sexual abuse, adult sexual abuse, adult sexual assault, and adult physical abuse. *Child Maltreatment, 5(1)*, 18-27.

Miller, M. (1999). A model to explain the relationship between sexual abuse and HIV risk among women. *AIDS Care, 11(1)*, 3-20.

Morrow, K. (1995). Lesbian women and HIV/AIDS. In A. O'Leary & L. Jemmott (Eds.), *Women at risk: Issues in the primary prevention of AIDS* (pp. 237-256). New York: Plenum Press.

Patterson, T., Semple, S., Temoshok, L., Atkinson, J., McCutchan, J., Straits-Troster, K., Chandler, J., & Grant, I. (1993). Depressive symptoms among HIV positive men: Life stress, coping, and social support. *Journal of Applied Behavioral Research, 1(1)*, 64-87.

Peterson, J., Folkman, S., & Bakeman, R. (1996). Stress, coping, HIV status, psychosocial resources, and depressive mood in African American gay, bisexual, and heterosexual men. *American Journal of Community Psychology, 24(4)*, 461-487.

Radloff, L. (1977). The CES-D Scale: A self-report depression scale for research in the general population. *Applied Psychological Measurement, 1(3)*, 385-401.

Roberts, S. & Sorensen, L. (1999). Prevalence of childhood sexual abuse and related sequelae in a lesbian population. *Journal of the Gay and Lesbian Medical Association, 3(1)*, 11-18.

Schwarzer, R., Dunkel-Schetter, C., & Kemeny, M. (1994). The multidimensional nature of received social support in gay men at risk of HIV infection and AIDS. *American Journal of Community Psychology, 22*, 319-339.

Simoni, J. M., & Ng, M. (2002). Abuse, health locus of control, and perceived health among HIV+ women. *Health Psychology, 21*, 89-93.

Simoni, J., Weinberg, B., & Nero, D. (1999). Training community members to conduct survey interviews: Notes from a study of seropositive women. *AIDS Education and Prevention, 11*, 87-88.

Stevens, P. (1993). Lesbians and HIV: Clinical, research, and policy issues. *American Journal of Orthopsychiatry, 63(2)*, 289-294.

Thompson, N., Potter, J., Sanderson, C., & Maibach, E. (1997). The relationship of sexual abuse and HIV risk behaviors among heterosexual adult female STD patients. *Child Abuse & Neglect, 21(2)*, 149-156.

Tjaden, P., Thoennes, N., & Allison, C. (1999). Comparing violence over the life span in sample of same-sex and opposite-sex cohabitants. *Violence and Victims, 14(4)*, 413-425.

Wyatt, G., Myers, H., Williams, J., Kitchen, C., Loeb, T., Carmona, J., Wyatt, L., Chin, D., & Presley, N. (2002). Does a history of trauma contribute to HIV risk for women of color? Implications for prevention and policy. *American Journal of Public Health, 92(4)*, 660-665.

Young, R., Friedman, S., Case, P., Asencio, M., & Clatts, M. (2000). Women injection drug users who have sex with women exhibit increased HIV infection and risk behaviors. *Journal of Drug Issues, 30(3)*, 499-524.

Lesbian and Bisexual Women's Experiences of Victimization: Mental Health, Revictimization, and Sexual Identity Development

Jessica F. Morris
Kimberly F. Balsam

SUMMARY. The prevalence and correlates of a variety of victimization experiences among a large, ethnically diverse national sample of 2,431 lesbian, bisexual, and gay women (LBG) is examined. Most participants (62.3%) report experiencing bias related victimization because

---

Jessica F. Morris, a licensed psychologist, received a PhD in Clinical Psychology from the University of Vermont and is a graduate of Vassar College. Her research and writing focus on the psychology of lesbians and have received a number of awards. In her clinical work, she specializes in psychological evaluations and community mental health; she also teaches psychology at the graduate level.

Kimberly F. Balsam received her PhD in Clinical Psychology from the University of Vermont and is currently a Postdoctoral Fellow at the University of Washington. Her research, teaching, and clinical interests focus on stress, trauma, and mental health among lesbian, gay, bisexual, and transgender populations.

Address correspondence to: Jessica F. Morris, P.O. Box 167, Sunderland, MA 01375.

The authors wish to thank Stacey Hart and Esther Rothblum for their helpful comments on earlier versions of this manuscript.

[Haworth co-indexing entry note]: "Lesbian and Bisexual Women's Experiences of Victimization: Mental Health, Revictimization, and Sexual Identity Development." Morris, Jessica F., and Kimberly F. Balsam. Co-published simultaneously in *Journal of Lesbian Studies* (Harrington Park Press, an imprint of The Haworth Press, Inc.) Vol. 7, No. 4, 2003, pp. 67-85; and: *Trauma, Stress, and Resilience Among Sexual Minority Women: Rising Like the Phoenix* (ed: Kimberly F. Balsam) Harrington Park Press, an imprint of The Haworth Press, Inc., 2003, pp. 67-85. Single or multiple copies of this article are available for a fee from The Haworth Document Delivery Service [1-800-HAWORTH, 9:00 a.m. - 5:00 p.m. (EST). E-mail address: docdelivery@haworthpress.com].

http://www.haworthpress.com/store/product.asp?sku=J155

10.1300/J155v07n04_05

they are LBG. Overall, 30.8% of participants report being harshly beaten or physically abused in childhood and 21.2% in adulthood; 39.3% report sexual victimization before the age of sixteen and 36.2% at age sixteen or older. Each type of victimization was significantly related to current psychological distress, and the more types of victimization (sexual or physical, in childhood or adulthood) a participant experienced, the greater her psychological distress. Participants who were victimized in childhood were four times more likely to experience the same type of victimization (sexual or physical) as an adult and about twice as likely to experience the other type of victimization in adulthood. In addition, there were significant differences in history of victimization by race/ethnicity. Native American participants reported the highest rates followed by Latinas, African Americans, Asian Americans, and Whites.

KEYWORDS. Trauma, physical abuse, sexual abuse, lesbian, bisexual, women of color, revictimization

Over the past two decades, there has been increased research focusing on violence against women. As a result, a robust body of literature exists demonstrating that women are frequently the victims of physical and sexual violence in their homes and communities; these victimization experiences have dire consequences for women's mental health over the lifespan. However, one important limitation of the violence against women literature is that it has largely focused on heterosexual women. Large-scale, national studies of childhood abuse, sexual assault, and domestic violence generally have not assessed sexual orientation, while smaller, convenience samples of lesbians often have not assessed for violence (Balsam, 2003).

Despite the relative lack of research in this area, the emerging picture suggests elevated rates of childhood physical abuse (Corliss, Cochran, & Mays, 2002), childhood sexual abuse (Hughes, Johnson, & Wilsnack, 2001; Roberts & Sorenson, 1999; Tjaden, Thoeness, & Allison, 1999; Tomeo, Templer, Anderson, & Kotler, 2001) and adult sexual assault (e.g., Duncan, 1990; Hughes et al., 2001; Tjaden et al., 1999; Tomeo et al., 2001) among lesbian and bisexual women as compared to heterosexual women. Furthermore, bias related victimization or hate crimes, particularly verbal abuse and harassment, have been reported by a majority of lesbians in large surveys (e.g., Herek, Gillis, Cogan, &

Glunt, 1997). Studies of domestic violence have yielded mixed results; some have found relatively low rates of domestic violence among lesbian and bisexual women (e.g., Descamps, Rothblum, Bradford, & Ryan, 2000), while others have found similar rates (see Burke & Follingstad, 1999, for a review) or even higher rates than for heterosexual women (e.g., Tjaden et al., 1999).

Despite some recent attention to lesbian and bisexual women's victimization, three important areas have yet to be addressed in the empirical literature. First, the existing studies generally focus on prevalence rates but do not examine the mental health correlates of victimization. Given that victimization is strongly associated with mental health problems in the general population of women, it is important to examine whether these associations differ among sexual minority women. Second, studies of the general population of women suggest that individuals who are victimized once have a greater risk of revictimization (e.g., Banyard, Williams, & Siegel, 2001), and that those who are multiply victimized report greater psychological distress than those with only one victimization experience (e.g., Messman-Moore, Long, & Siegfried, 2000). While a few studies have documented similar phenomena among lesbians (e.g., Descamps et al., 2000; Lockhart, White, Causby, & Isaac, 1994; Tuel & Russell, 1998), the majority of studies do not examine both physical and sexual abuse in childhood and adulthood, nor do they include general measures of mental health or psychological distress. Third, the study of victimization, both among the general population of women and among lesbians, has generally focused on white women's experiences; little is known about victimization and mental health in the lives of women of color. Greene (1994) explains that lesbians of color face a "triple jeopardy," with gender, ethnicity, and sexual orientation as potentially disempowering statuses. Thus, this group of women may be particularly vulnerable to physical and sexual victimization.

One of the potential reasons for the dearth of literature on LBG women and trauma is the widespread cultural myth that victimization may "cause a woman to become a lesbian." In particular, childhood sexual abuse is often assumed to be a "causal" factor in sexual identity development (Balsam, 2003; Butke, 1995; Hall, 1998). Researchers may have avoided this area out of the fear that their results would be used to support such potentially damaging myths and stereotypes. Thus, while there is no evidence to support these myths, we know little about how sexual identity development is impacted by childhood experiences of sexual abuse. Given that adult expression of sexuality has been found to be affected by childhood sexual assault (e.g., Briere, 1992), it is reasonable to assume that this would be the case for LBG women as well. For example, early sexual victimization might force a girl to become aware of her sexual feelings at an early age, and thus "come out" as a lesbian earlier. Alternatively, such victimization may cause her to learn to "numb" or dissociate from her feelings

(Briere, 1992) and thus she may take longer to develop awareness of her sexual orientation. In the face of cultural myths about sexual abuse "causing" LBG orientation, a woman might fear that her same-sex attractions are merely a "symptom" of abuse she experienced by men, and thus experience greater distress and confusion in the development of a healthy sexual identity. While these questions have been raised in the clinical and theoretical literature (e.g., Balsam, 2003; Butke, 1995), they have not been examined empirically in a sample of lesbian and bisexual women.

The present study used a large data set of 2,431 participants who filled out a "Lesbian Wellness Survey" in 1994-1995 (Morris, Balsam, & Rothblum, 2001; Morris & Rothblum, 1999; Morris, Waldo, & Rothblum, 2001). In contrast to the respondents in other large-scale studies of sexual minority women, 25% of the lesbians and bisexual women in this data set were women of color. The survey contained sections that asked about experiences with violence, including adult and childhood physical and sexual abuse. Thus, it is possible to provide descriptive data regarding experiences of victimization over the lifespan, as well as to explore the degree and impact of revictimization and multiple victimization in a sample of lesbian and bisexual women. In addition, the diversity of race and ethnicity of the sample allowed us to examine victimization factors for African American, Latina, Native American, Asian American, and European American women, separately. The data set included a measure of mental health, allowing us to examine the degree to which different types of victimization impact psychological functioning. Furthermore, questions about milestones in the coming out process provide an opportunity to examine the relationship between childhood sexual abuse and sexual identity development.

The purpose of this paper is to examine the prevalence and correlates of a variety of victimization experiences among a large, ethnically diverse national sample of lesbian and bisexual women. While lesbian and bisexual women may experience specific risks for victimization and poor mental health outcome, it is also likely that they experience strengths or resilience factors due to their sexual orientation that may protect against or moderate the negative mental health consequences of victimization (Balsam, 2003). Therefore, the study will examine the extent to which childhood and adulthood physical and sexual abuse predict current levels of psychological distress. Revictimization, the degree to which experiences of childhood physical and sexual abuse predict adult experiences of domestic violence, sexual assault, and anti-LBG victimization for lesbian and bisexual women will be explored. In this study, lesbian and bisexual women who report having been sexually abused in childhood will be compared with those who do not report such abuse on dimensions of sexual identity development, including ages at which they reached the various coming out milestones and degree of outness.

METHOD

Participants

The data set consisted of 2,431 women from every U.S. state. In 1994-1995, 10,000 questionnaires were distributed to feminist, gay, and lesbian bookstores and community centers; lesbian and gay political and social groups; lesbian and gay national mailing lists; and friendship networks. In addition, advertisements about the study were placed in feminist and lesbian periodicals.

Procedure

The "Lesbian Wellness Survey" was described as "a survey by lesbians for any woman who has loved other women." The purpose was to understand "what lives are like for lesbian and bisexual women in the U.S." Questionnaires were completed without names or addresses, and mailed back in postage-paid return envelopes. There were five respondents who were not included in the analyses because they indicated both exclusively heterosexual identity and sexual experience only with men.

Measures

Demographic variables. The Lesbian Wellness Survey included items about age, race/ethnicity, size of city/town, religion while growing up and current religion, frequency of attending religious services, employment status, occupation, education, annual income, household composition, and current and past relationship status.

Violence variables. The questionnaire asked respondents about their experiences with violence throughout their life. One question asked "Have you ever been harshly beaten or physically abused" and respondents were asked to provide answers both for "while growing up" and "as an adult" for a list of specific people. These people were male relative, female relative, male acquaintance, female acquaintance, male stranger, and female stranger; for the adult section female lover, husband, and other male lover were also included. Another question asked "Before the age of 16 did any relative force you to engage in sexual activities" and listed the following relatives: father, mother, grandfather, grandmother, uncle, aunt, brother, sister, stepfather, stepmother, foster father, foster mother, male cousin, and female cousin. Separate questions asked, "Before the age of 16 did any stranger (person you didn't know) force you to engage in sexual activities" and about acquaintances or friends, "Before the age of 16 did someone you knew who was not a relative force you to engage in sexual activities." There were also questions about adulthood: "When you were 16 or older did anyone force you to engage in sexual activities" and listed male relative, male acquaintance, male stranger, female relative, female acquaintance, female stranger, male lover/boyfriend/husband, and female lover/girlfriend/partner.

Anti-LBG victimization. Experiences with hate crimes and anti-LBG victimization were asked about with "Have any of the following happened to you because you are lesbian/bisexual/gay" and listed specific types of experiences: verbally attacked or harassed, lost job, home or property damage, physically attacked, sexual assault, rape, and discharged from military. There were four additional bias-related questions that were asked only of those participants who had children. These questions were: (a) "Threatened with loss of custody of a child," (b) "Actually lost custody of a child," (c) "Harassed/threatened/discriminated against by your children's school or other parents," and (d) "Have your children been harassed/threatened/discriminated against because you are lesbian/bisexual/gay."

Aspects of the lesbian/bisexual experience. Sexual orientation was measured on a continuous line from "exclusively lesbian/gay" to "exclusively heterosexual" with "bisexual" at the midpoint. This item was scored from 0 to 100 by use of a template, with lower scores indicating lesbian identity.

Sexual experience was defined as the proportion of sexual experience with women versus men. The item was phrased, "In terms of your consensual sexual behavior since you became sexually active, where would you put yourself on this line?" The item was measured on a continuous line from "only women" to "only men" with "equally both sexes" as the midpoint, and scored from 0 to 100 by use of a template. Lower scores indicated a greater proportion of female versus male sexual experiences.

Outness/disclosure consisted of the percentage of family, lesbian/bisexual/gay (LBG) friends, heterosexual friends, and coworkers whom participants had informed that they were LBG. This subscale was adapted from the National Lesbian Health Care Survey (Bradford, Ryan, & Rothblum, 1994) and resulted in a total outness/disclosure score.

Milestones in the coming out process included items about ages at which respondents first (a) questioned that they might be LBG, (b) thought of themselves as LBG, (c) told someone that they were LBG, (d) had a sexual experience with another woman, (e) told their mother they were LBG, (f) told their father they were LBG, and (g) told a sibling they were LBG.

Mental health. Overall severity and prevalence of psychological distress was measured with the Brief Symptom Inventory (BSI), which is a 53-item scale designed to measure a variety of psychological symptoms (Derogatis &

Spencer, 1982). The Global Severity Index (GSI) comprises all 53 items of the BSI and is an overall measure of psychological distress. Each item represents one problem and respondents rate how much discomfort they have felt as a result of that problem over the last week on a five-point scale from 0 ("not at all") to 4 ("extremely"). The GSI has test-retest reliability coefficient of .90. The internal consistency of the BSI for this sample was a Cronbach's alpha of .96.

RESULTS

Demographic information. The 2,431 participants in this study are a large and diverse group; the average age is 36 with a range from 15-83. The majority of participants, 75% (n = 1823) are White/Caucasian, 10% (n = 238) are African American/Black, 7% (n = 177) are Latina, 4% (n = 89) are Native American/American Indian, 3% (n = 64) are Asian American/Pacific Islander, and 2% (n = 40) indicated "other" or did not respond. Overall, participants report a high level of education; approximately three-fourths have a college degree or higher. Most participants, 70%, report being employed full time, 17% part time, 7% unemployed, and 24% are students (the categories are not mutually exclusive). The participants report a low range of yearly incomes, with 38% earning under $20,000 per year, 52% earning between $20,000 and $49,000, and the remaining 10% earning $50,000 and over. Participants are from every state in the United States, and are equally distributed throughout the regions of the United States. Approximately one-quarter are from each region: Northeast, Southeast, Midwest, and West. In terms of the type of geographic location, the majority are from urban areas: 28% large city, 29% medium city, 24% small city or town, 10% suburb, 8% rural, and 1% did not respond or indicated "other" (such as in prison).

The majority of participants (65%) report that they are in a primary relationship with a woman, and 26% are single. Smaller portions of participants report dating women casually (11%), dating both women and men (2%), dating men casually (1%), and being in a primary relationship with a man (5%). Participants' living situations reflect their relationship status, with 48% living with their female partner/lover, 28% living alone, and the rest living in a variety of other situations such as with housemates, children, or parents. Twenty-seven percent of participants report ever being legally married to a man and 41% say they had a primary relationship with a man in the past. In addition, 21% of participants report having children.

Aspects of the lesbian/bisexual experience. Sexual orientation ranges from 0 (exclusively lesbian) to 100 (exclusively heterosexual). The average score on this item is 13, with 44% of respondents self-identifying as exclusively lesbian (scored as 0), 18% in the range between 1 and 10, 8% between 11 and 20, 26% between 21 and 50, and 3% between 51 and 100. Sexual experience also ranges from 0-100 (0 = only women, 100 = only men), with an average of 25, indicating that most of the respondents' relationships are and have been with women. The outness/disclosure variable ranges from 0-100 with a mean overall score of 71.31, indicating the sample is out to just under three-quarters of family, friends, and coworkers.

On average, participants first questioned being LBG at 17.7 years old, had a first sexual experience with a woman at 21.8, and first thought of themselves as LBG at 22.5; 2% say they have not had a sexual experience with a woman. Participants were 23.6 years old on average when they first told someone they wer LGB.

Anti-LBG victimization. Overall, 62.3% of participants report experiencing a hate crime or bias victimization because they are LBG and 41.3% report only one type of experience. The most common, by far, is being verbally attacked or harassed because they are LBG, which 56.6% of participants report. Many fewer participants report loss of employment (9.2%), home or property damage (9.0%), or physical attack (6.5%). Less than two percent report either sexual assault, rape, or being discharged from the military based on their sexual orientation. Some participants who had children reported being harassed, threatened, or discriminated against by the children's school (16.2% of mothers) or that their children experienced harassment, threats, or discrimination because of the mother's sexual orientation (21.5% of mothers).

Physical abuse. About one-third (30.8%) of participants report being harshly beaten or physically abused in childhood and 21.2% in adulthood. Table 1 shows the types of perpetrators of physical violence reported by participants. For violence in intimate relationships, about the same percent of participants report being beaten by a female lover/partner (9.2%) as a male lover/husband (9.3%). However, most participants who where beaten by a lover report both male and female perpetrators (7.7%).

Sexual assault. Overall, 53.1% of participants report some sort of sexual victimization in their past. Specifically, 39.3% report being sexually assaulted by someone before the age of sixteen and 36.2% report being sexually assaulted by someone when they were sixteen or older. Looking at multiple victimization, 21.6% report sexual assault both before and after age sixteen and 32.3% report either before or after age sixteen but not both. Table 2 presents the details of which relatives were perpetrators. Table 3 presents the details of sexual assault from age sixteen or older by perpetrators.

Violence variables. The types of violence were summarized into four dichotomous (yes/no) variables: (a) sexually assaulted by any perpetrator in childhood, (b) physically abused by any perpetrator in childhood, (c) sexually

TABLE 1. Percent of Participants (N = 2431) Who Report Being Harshly Beaten or Physically Abused While Growing Up or as an Adult

	While growing up	As an adult
Male relative	22.1	2.2
Female relative	15.7	1.2
Male acquaintance	4.9	3.2
Female acquaintance	2.1	1.8
Male stranger	2.5	3.1
Female stranger	0.6	0.7
Female lover	N/A	9.2
Husband, other male lover	N/A	9.3
At least one perpetrator	30.8	21.2

TABLE 2. Type of Perpetrator Forcing Participants to Engage in Sexual Activities Before Age Sixteen

	Percent
Father	7.4
Mother	2.1
Grandfather	2.9
Grandmother	0.6
Uncle	6.2
Aunt	0.5
Brother	6.3
Sister	0.5
Stepfather	2.9
Stepmother	0.1
Foster Father	0.3
Foster Mother [a]	0.0
Male Cousin	5.4
Female Cousin	0.6
Sexual abuse by any relative	25.7
Stranger	13.3
Acquaintance	23.7
Sexual abuse by anyone	39.3

[a] n = 1

assaulted by any perpetrator in adulthood, and (d) physically abused by any perpetrator in adulthood. A "multiple trauma" summary variable was calculated from these four summary variables with five levels: no abuse reported or one, two, three, or all four types reported. The results of this multiple trauma variable show that 36.6% of participants did not report any type of physical or sexual abuse; 25% reported one type, 19.9% report two types, 11.3% reported three types, and 7.2% reported all four.

Victimization and mental health. An analysis of variance was conducted with psychological distress (GSI scale from the BSI) predicted from the four dichotomous variables created: reported sexual assault and/or physical abuse in childhood and/or in adulthood. Overall, the ANOVA was significant, $F(4, 2419) = 59.180$, $p < .001$ and accounted for 8.9% of variance in psychological distress. Each of the variables–sexual assault as a child, sexual assault as an adult, physical abuse as a child, and physical abuse as an adult–was uniquely significant in predicting current psychological distress. In a separate analysis, the multiple trauma variable showed a significant correlation with the GSI score, $r = .30$, $p < .001$, suggesting that the more types of victimization a participant experienced, the greater her psychological distress.

Revictimization. Revictimization was a common experience reported by participants. Assault or abuse in childhood was a predictor of adult experiences of victimization. Specifically, participants who reported being sexually assaulted by any perpetrator during childhood were significantly more likely to report sexual assault as an adult (55.0%) than those who were not sexual as-

TABLE 3. Type of Perpetrator Forcing Participants to Engage in Sexual Activities at Age Sixteen or Older

	Percent
Male lover, boyfriend, husband	13.3
Female lover, girlfriend, partner	3.5
Male acquaintance	18.6
Male stranger	10.4
Male relative	6.5
Female acquaintance	2.1
Female relative	0.9
Female stranger	0.7
Sexual abuse by any male	34.3
Sexual abuse by any female	5.8
Sexual abuse by anyone	36.2

saulted as children (24.0%), $\chi^2 = 241.7$, $p < .001$. Those sexually assaulted in childhood were also significantly more likely to report physical abuse as an adult (30.3%) than those who were not sexually assaulted as children (15.2%), $\chi^2 = 79.7$, $p < .001$. Participants who reported being physically abused by any perpetrator in childhood were significantly more likely to report physical abuse as an adult (39.4%) than those who were not physically abused as children (13.0%), $\chi^2 = 216.4$, $p < .001$. Those physically abused in childhood were also significantly more likely to report sexual assault as an adult (52.9%) than those who were not physically abused as children (47.1%), $\chi^2 = 130.8$, $p < .001$. Those who were victimized in childhood are about four times more likely to experience the same type of victimization (sexual or physical) as an adult and about twice as likely to experience the other type of victimization in adulthood.

Aspects of lesbian identity and history of childhood sexual assault. Participants who reported being sexually assaulted as children by any perpetrator differ in significant ways, from those who were not sexually assaulted, on some of the dimensions of lesbian identity and the milestones in the coming out process, $F\,(7, 2252) = 4.846$, $p < .001$ (Table 4 shows the means for each group). However, participants with a childhood sexual assault history did not differ from participants without such a history on the proportion of *consensual* sexual experiences with women and men since becoming sexually active, sexual orientation identity (a continuum of lesbian, bisexual, and heterosexual), or degree of outness. But, participants did significantly differ on ages at which they reached milestones in the coming-out process. Specifically, participants with a history of childhood sexual abuse reported first being aware of being LBG, first self-identifying as LBG, and having their first same-sex sexual experience at earlier ages than those without such a history.

TABLE 4. Age at Which Participants Reached Milestones in the Coming Out Process by Childhood Sexual Assault History

	Yes childhood sexual assault	No childhood sexual assault
First questioned being LBG**	16.9	18.1
First consensual sex with a woman**	20.9	22.3
First thought of self as LBG*	21.9	22.7
First told someone you are LBG	23.2	23.7

Note: *$p < .05$, **$p < .001$.

It is interesting to note that many participants who reported a history of childhood sexual assault wrote comments stating that they were not lesbians "because of" the sexual assault. These participants emphasized that they did not want the researchers to hypothesize a causal relationship between childhood sexual assault and adult LBG identity.

Differences by race/ethnicity. In order to examine the relationship between race/ethnicity and victimization, white participants and women of color were compared on the multiple trauma variable, which was a summary variable representing no abuse reported or one, two, three, or all four types reported (and scored from 0 to 4). Native American participants reported the highest trauma level of 2.14 followed by Latina, 1.67; African American, 1.42; Asian American, 1.17; and White, 1.16. There was an overall significant difference in trauma level by race $F(4, 2389) = 19.904, p < .001$. Multiple comparisons revealed which groups were significantly different and these data are presented in Table 5. The trauma level variable was a summary of types of victimization. For more detailed information, Figure 1 presents each of these victimization experiences for the different racial/ethnic groups.

DISCUSSION

Although violence against women has gained the attention of many social science researchers, few studies have specifically examined lesbian and bisexual women's experiences of victimization. The current study adds to our knowledge base by providing information from a large, ethnically diverse sample about lesbian and bisexual women's experiences of physical and sexual violence in childhood and adulthood, as well as experiences of bias motivated verbal and physical victimization. The most common experience was

TABLE 5. Significance of Differences in Multiple Trauma Variable by Race

	African American	Asian American	Latina	Native American	White
White	$p < .01$	N.S.	$p < .001$	$p < .001$	
Native American	$p < .001$	$p < .001$	$p < .01$		
Latina	$p < .05$	$p < .01$			
Asian American	N.S.				
Multiple Trauma	1.42	1.17	1.67	2.14	1.16

Note: For the multiple trauma variable, higher numbers indicate more types of trauma.

FIGURE 1. Percent of Participants Reporting Experiences with Types of Victimization by Race/Ethnicity

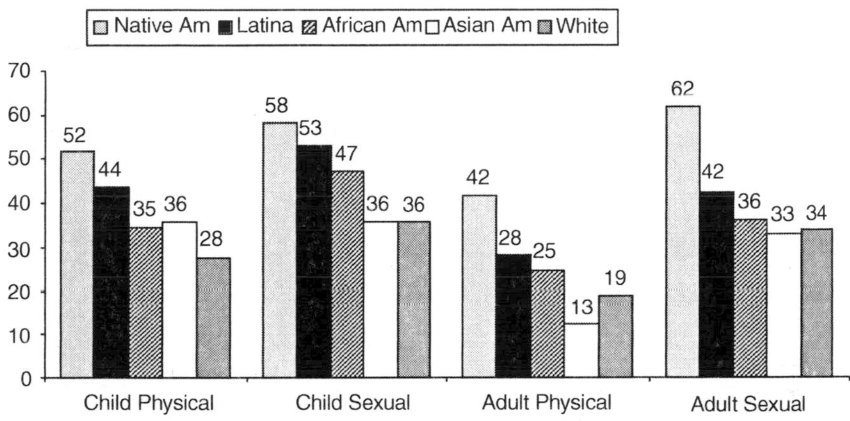

anti-LBG verbal harassment reported by over half the women; about three out of five participants reported any type of bias-related victimization. One in five mothers reported their children had been verbally harassed because of the mother's sexual orientation (see also Morris, Balsam, & Rothblum, 2001). Overall, the majority of participants report some sort of victimization experience due to their sexual orientation. This is one form of violence that lesbians experience because of their sexual orientation, and therefore it is not comparable to the experiences of heterosexual women. These results concur with Neisen's (1993) assertion that lesbians and bisexual women must contend, on an ongoing basis, with "cultural victimization," the continuing stress of living with homophobia and heterosexism. Thus, any other experiences of physical or sexual victimization must be understood in the context of these ongoing stressors.

About three out of five participants reported some form of physical or sexual victimization at least once in their life. These results suggest that lesbians, despite certain protective factors, are at least as vulnerable to violence as women in the general population. Prevalence rates for physical and sexual victimization in the general population of women vary widely according to methodological issues such as age cutoffs, sampling strategies and, most importantly, the wording of the questions (Silvern, Waedle, Baughan, Karyl, & Kaersvang, 2000; Russell & Bolen, 2000). The rates found in the current study fall towards the high end of the ranges generally reported in large-scale surveys of women. This may indicate that lesbian and bisexual women are, in fact, at greater risk for victimization. Future studies should examine this question using comparison groups of heterosexual women. It must also be considered that the current study used subjective questions to assess victimization. In contrast to clearly-defined behavioral measures, such questions require participants to define their experiences as "victimization" or "abuse." Subjective measures generally yield lower prevalence estimates than behaviorally-defined measures (Silvern et al., 2000). However, it may be that lesbian and bisexual women are particularly likely to self-define experiences as "abuse." The influence of feminist values on the LBG community, greater use of psychotherapy (Corliss, Cochran, & Mays, 2002; Rothblum & Factor, 2001), and cultural norms within the LBG community could potentially contribute to a tendency to acknowledge and report experiences as abuse, potentially inflating the rates found in this study. Such issues should be further examined in future research.

Of the violence experienced by participants, more was reported in childhood than adulthood. Childhood sexual assault was reported by about four in ten participants, while childhood physical abuse was reported by about three in ten participants. These prevalence estimates are high; future research should examine potential factors that might account for lesbian and bisexual women's risk for victimization in childhood, particularly given that this victimization most likely occurred before these women were "out" to themselves and others. Furthermore, the mediators of risk may be different for different types of abuse. Perpetrators of physical abuse were most likely to be relatives whereas sexual assault perpetrators were as likely to be acquaintances as relatives. While most of the perpetrators of both types of violence were male, some women did report either physical abuse or sexual assault by female perpetrators in childhood.

Two in ten participants reported physical abuse in adulthood and just under four in ten reported sexual assault in adulthood. It was within intimate relationships that most incidents of physical abuse occurred. Equal numbers of participants (9% of the total sample) reported experiencing physical violence by male versus female partners. Previous large-scale studies of domestic violence among lesbians (e.g., Descamps et al., 2000) have not assessed the gender of the perpetrator. The current study adds to our understanding of domestic violence experienced by lesbian and bisexual women and suggests that these women are equally at risk in their intimate relationships with men and with women. Another intriguing result of the current study is that the majority of participants who reported any physical violence by a partner reported both male and female perpetrators. Thus, it may be that the factors that place a woman at risk for partner violence are present, regardless of whether she is currently in a relationship with a man or a woman. In contrast, most of the sexual victimization reported was committed by male perpetrators. Similar to findings in studies of heterosexual women (Koss, Gidycz, & Wisniewski, 1987), male acquaintances and male partners were the most common perpetrators of such abuse.

Other than the National Lesbian Health Care Survey (Bradford, Ryan, & Rothblum, 1994), no research has examined the degree to which lifetime victimization among lesbian and bisexual women is associated with their current psychological distress. This study found that each type of abuse assessed–physical abuse in childhood, physical abuse in adulthood, sexual assault in childhood, and sexual assault in adulthood–uniquely predicted participants' current psychological distress. Additionally, the rates of revictimization in this study demonstrate that those who are victimized in childhood are more likely to report being victimized in adulthood, results that mirror those found with the general population of women (Gidycz, Coble, Latham, & Layman, 1993). These experiences of multiple victimization were associated with even greater psychological distress among participants. Thus, findings with regards to mental health and revictimization suggest some similarities among women across sexual orientation groups.

Alternatively, unlike heterosexual women, lesbian and bisexual women who experience sexual abuse must contend with the cultural myths regarding the impact of abuse on sexual identity. In the current study, some participants expressed concern about their lesbian identity development being seen as a reaction to negative experiences with men, especially childhood sexual abuse. While it was not the purpose of this study to examine this directly, the results suggest that LBG identity development was in some ways unrelated to childhood sexual abuse. No difference was found–based upon whether the participant reported childhood sexual abuse or not–in either sexual identity (more lesbian versus more heterosexual) or in proportion of consensual sexual behavior with women versus men. Nor was there a difference in the age at which a participant first disclosed her sexual identity to another person. However, participants who reported childhood sexual abuse did report questioning and thinking of self as being LBG, as well as engaging in their first sexual experience with another woman, at earlier ages than those without sexual abuse histories. It may be that women who are aware of their orientation at earlier ages engage in more behaviors that put them at risk for victimization. Additionally, the experience of sexual abuse may heighten these girls' awareness of their sexuality at earlier ages, thus forcing them to examine their attractions and identity at earlier ages than their peers.

This study is the first to report data concerning rates of victimization among different ethnic/racial groups of lesbian and bisexual women. There were significant differences based on race, with Asian American and white participants reporting lower rates of victimization than other participants. Native American women reported the highest rates, followed by Latina and African American women. Since this area of research is so new, it is difficult to know whether these results are particular to the participants in this study or reflect more common differences in the population. Root (1996) suggests that women of color's multiply marginalized status may leave them particularly vulnerable to victimization. Lesbian and bisexual women, who must contend with homophobia as well as racism and sexism, could conceivably experience even greater vulnerability. Importantly, however, the current study suggests the importance of recruiting large enough numbers to examine different ethnic/racial groups of lesbian and bisexual women separately, rather than grouping together all of the women of color into a single category. It will be important for future researchers to examine more closely the social and cultural factors that may be associated with ethnic/racial differences in victimization risk.

With over 2,400 participants, this project is one of the largest studies of participants completing a "lesbian" questionnaire ever conducted. Further, it has more demographic diversity than any other research focusing on the lesbian experience. This study has similar limitations to questionnaire studies in general, and those using self-identified lesbian and bisexual participants in particular. The participants were a convenience, not random, sample, and therefore the results cannot be generalized to all lesbian and bisexual women in the United States. As with all self-report survey data, these data need to be interpreted carefully. Further, retrospective self-report of childhood experiences can be less accurate than self-report of current experiences. However, it has been suggested that women who answer surveys about lesbian and bisexual issues may be representative of those who psychologists and other mental health or medical professionals are most likely encounter as clients, patients, or research participants (Rothblum, 1994). Thus, it may be possible to generalize from these self-report survey findings to those U.S. lesbian and bisexual women for whom mental health or medical professionals provide services.

These results may be helpful to mental health practitioners in that they suggest lesbian and bisexual women are, overall, somewhat similar to heterosexual women in their experiences with victimization. As with women in general, victimization experiences of lesbian and bisexual women have significant bearing on their mental health. Thus, the clinical literature on treating survivors of victimization may be at least somewhat applicable in treating lesbian and bisexual survivors who seek assistance. The prevalence rates found in this sample certainly suggest that practitioners should routinely screen for victimization histories of lesbian and bisexual clients, both in childhood and adulthood. Practitioners should be particularly sensitive to the issue of violence in the lives of lesbians and bisexual women of color.

In addition to similarities with heterosexual women, these results also highlight some of the unique aspects of victimization in the lives of lesbian and bisexual women. One important difference is that LBG women experience adult abuse, both sexual and physical, from female perpetrators, including within intimate relationships. A large proportion of women who reported adult physical abuse said they had both female and male perpetrators. Therapists working with women who previously experienced violence within their relationships with men are advised to be aware that this pattern maybe repeated, even if the client is now in relationships with women. Therefore, therapists should not make the assumption that these women are now "safe" from additional domestic violence because they are currently in relationships with women rather than men. Furthermore, lesbian and bisexual women are uniquely vulnerable to bias- related harassment and hate crimes, which can have particularly deleterious effects on mental health (Herek, Gillis, & Cogan, 1999). Additionally, the findings with regards to sexual identity development suggest the potential importance of exploring the relationship between childhood sexual abuse and the coming out process with lesbian and bisexual survivors.

REFERENCES

Balsam, K. F. (2003). Traumatic victimization in the lives of lesbian and bisexual women: A contextual approach. *Journal of Lesbian Studies, 7(1)*, 1-14.

Banyard, V. L., Williams, L. M., & Siegel, J. A. (2001). Understanding links among childhood trauma, dissociation, and women's mental health. *American Journal of Orthopsychiatry, 71*, 311-321.

Bradford, J., Ryan, C., & Rothblum, E. D. (1994). National lesbian health care survey: Implications for mental health. *Journal of Consulting and Clinical Psychology, 62*, 228-242.

Briere, J. (1992). *Child abuse trauma: Theory and treatment of the lasting effects.* Newbury Park, CA: Sage.

Burke, L. K. & Follingstad, D. R. (1999). Violence in lesbian and gay relationships: Theory, prevalence, and correlational factors. *Clinical Psychology Review, 19(5)*, 487-512.

Butke, M. (1995). Lesbians and sexual child abuse. In L.A. Fuentes (Ed.) *Sexual abuse in nine North American cultures* (pp. 236-258). Thousand Oaks, CA: Sage.

Corliss, H. L., Cochran, S. D., & Mays, V. M. (2002). Reports of parental maltreatment during childhood in a United States population-based survey of homosexual, bisexual, and heterosexual adults. *Child Abuse & Neglect, 26*, 1165-1178.

Derogatis, L. R. & Spencer, P. M. (1982). *Brief symptom inventory (BSI): Administration, scoring, & procedures manual–I.* Baltimore, MD: Author.

Descamps, M. J., Rothblum, E. D., Bradford, J., & Ryan, C. (2000). Mental health impact of child sexual abuse, rape, intimate partner violence, and hate crimes in the National Lesbian Health Care Survey. *Journal of Gay & Lesbian Social Services, 11*, 27-55.

Greene, B. (1994). Lesbian women of color: Triple jeopardy. In L. Comas-Diaz & B. Greene (Eds.), *Women of color: Integrating ethnic and gender identities in psychotherapy* (pp. 389-427). NY: Guilford.

Hall, J. (1998). Lesbians surviving childhood sexual abuse: Pivotal experiences related to sexual orientation, gender, and race. *Journal of Lesbian Studies, 2(1)*, 7-28.

Herek, G. M., Gillis, J. R., & Cogan, J. C. (1999). Psychological sequelae of hate crime victimization among lesbian, gay, and bisexual adults. *Journal of Consulting and Clinical Psychology, 6*, 945-951.

Herek, G. M., Gillis, J. R., Cogan, J. C., & Glunt, E. K. (1997). Hate crime victimization among lesbian, gay, and bisexual adults. *Journal of Interpersonal Violence, 12(2)*, 195-215.

Hughes, T. L., Johnson, T., & Wilsnack, S. C. (2001). Sexual assault and alcohol abuse: A comparison of lesbians and heterosexual women. *Journal of Substance Abuse, 13*, 515-532.

Koss, M. P., Gidycz, C. A., & Wisniewski, N. (1987). The scope of rape: Incidence and prevalence of sexual aggression and victimization in a national sample of higher education students. *Journal of Consulting and Clinical Psychology, 55*, 162-170.

Lockhart, L. L., White, B. W., Causby, V., & Isaac, A. (1994). Letting out the secret: Violence in lesbian relationships. *Journal of Interpersonal Violence, 9(4)*, 469-492.

Messman-Moore, T. L., Long, P. J., & Siegfried, N. J. (2000). The revictimization of child sexual abuse survivors: An examination of the adjustment of college women with child sexual abuse, adult sexual assault, and adult physical abuse. *Child Maltreatment, 5(1)*, 18-27.

Morris, J. F., Balsam, K. F., & Rothblum, E. D. (2002). A comparison of lesbians and bisexual mothers and non-mothers: Demographics and milestones in the coming out process. *Journal of Family Psychology, 16(2)*, 144-156.

Morris, J. F. & Rothblum, E. D. (1999). Who fills out a lesbian questionnaire: Years out, disclosure of sexual orientation, sexual experience with women, and participation in the lesbian community. *Psychology of Women Quarterly, 23*, 537-557.

Morris, J. F., Waldo, C. R., & Rothblum, E. D. (2001). A model of predictors and outcomes of outness among lesbian and bisexual women. *American Journal of Orthopsychiatry, 71*, 61-71.

Neisen, J. H. (1993). Healing from cultural victimization: Recovery from shame due to heterosexism. *Journal of Gay & Lesbian Psychotherapy, 2(1)*, 49-63.

Roberts, S. J. & Sorensen, L. (1999). Health related behaviors and cancer screening of lesbians: Results from the Boston Lesbian Health Project. *Women & Health, 28(4)*, 1-12.

Root, M. P. P. (1996). Women of Color and traumatic stress in "domestic captivity": Gender and race as disempowering statuses. In A. J. Marsella, M. J. Friedman, E. T. Gerrity, & R. M. Scurfied (Eds.), *Ethnocultural aspects of Posttraumatic Stress Disorder* (pp. 363-388). Washington, D.C.: American Psychological Association.

Rothblum, E. D. (1994). I only read about myself on bathroom walls: The need for research on the mental health of lesbians and gay men. *Journal of Consulting and Clinical Psychology*, *62*, 213-220.

Rothblum, E. D., & Factor, R. J. (2001). Lesbians and their sisters as a control group: Demographic and mental health factors. *Psychological Science*, *12(1)*, 63-69.

Russell, D. E. H., & Bolen, R. M. (2000). *The epidemic of rape and child sexual abuse in the United States*. Thousand Oaks, CA: Sage.

Silvern, L., Waelde, L. C., Baughan, B. M., Karyl, J., & Kaersvang, L. L. (2000). Two formats for eliciting retrospective reports of child sexual and physical abuse: Effects on apparent prevalence and relationships to adjustment. *Child Maltreatment*, *5(3)*, 236-250.

Tjaden, P., Thoeness, N., & Allison, C. J. (1999). Comparing violence over the life span in samples of same-sex and opposite-sex cohabitants. *Violence and Victims*, *14(4)*, 413-425.

Tomeo, M. E., Templer, D. I., Anderson, S., & Kotler, D. (2001). Comparative data of childhood and adolescent molestation in heterosexual and homosexual persons. *Archives of Sexual Behavior*, *30*, 535-541.

Tuell, B. D. & Russell, R. K. (1998). Self-esteem and depression in battered women: A comparison of lesbian and heterosexual survivors. *Violence Against Women*, *4(3)*, 344-362.

Triple Jeopardy and Beyond: Multiple Minority Stress and Resilience Among Black Lesbians

Lisa Bowleg
Jennifer Huang
Kelly Brooks
Amy Black
Gary Burkholder

Lisa Bowleg, PhD, is a social psychologist and Assistant Professor in the Department of Psychology, University of Rhode Island.

Jennifer Huang, MA, is a doctoral candidate in the Experimental Psychology program at the University of Rhode Island.

Kelly Brooks is a doctoral student in the Experimental Psychology program at the University of Rhode Island.

Amy Black is a doctoral student in the Experimental Psychology program at the University of Rhode Island.

Gary Burkholder earned a PhD in Experimental Psychology from the University of Rhode Island. He currently works at the Brown University Institute for Community Health Promotion as a community health researcher. He also teaches social psychology and quantitative methods at Rhode Island School of Design and for Walden University.

The authors are grateful for the support of their research assistants, Babajide Adegoke, John DesRochers, Patricia DosSantos, Oswald Garrington, Michelle O'Connor, and Donna Taraborelli. The authors also appreciate the assistance of Melynda Craig, Department of Psychology, University of Rhode Island, who conducted the external audit of the study. Last, but not least, the authors are grateful to United Lesbians of African Heritage and the women who trusted them with their candor and narratives.

Address correspondence to: Lisa Bowleg, Department of Psychology, University of Rhode Island, 10 Woodward Hall, Kingston, RI 02881-0808 (E-mail: bowlegl@uri.edu).

[Haworth co-indexing entry note]: "Triple Jeopardy and Beyond: Multiple Minority Stress and Resilience Among Black Lesbians." Bowleg, Lisa et al. Co-published simultaneously in *Journal of Lesbian Studies* (Harrington Park Press, an imprint of The Haworth Press, Inc.) Vol. 7, No. 4, 2003, pp. 87-108; and: *Trauma, Stress, and Resilience Among Sexual Minority Women: Rising Like the Phoenix* (ed: Kimberly F. Balsam) Harrington Park Press, an imprint of The Haworth Press, Inc., 2003, pp. 87-108. Single or multiple copies of this article are available for a fee from The Haworth Document Delivery Service [1-800-HAWORTH, 9:00 a.m. - 5:00 p.m. (EST). E-mail address: docdelivery@haworthpress.com].

http://www.haworthpress.com/store/product.asp?sku=J155

10.1300/J155v07n04_06

SUMMARY. This qualitative study explored the experiences of multiple minority stress and resilience among interviewees at a retreat for Black lesbians. Participants were a predominantly middle-class, highly educated sample of Black women (*N* = 19) between the ages of 26 and 68. The multicultural model of stress (Slavin, Rainer, McCreary, & Gowda, 1991) and the transactional model of resilience (Kumpfer, 1999) were theoretical frameworks for the study. Most of the participants discussed racism as a mundane and significant stressor, and contextualized their experiences of sexism and heterosexism through the prism of racism. Study findings provide empirical support for the "triple jeopardy" experience of Black lesbians (Greene, 1995), as well as the six predictors of resilience in Kumpfer's (1999) transactional model of resilience.

KEYWORDS. Resilience, black lesbians, multiple minority stress, mundane stress

More than three decades ago, Beale (1970) described the experience of Black[1] women living in a racist and sexist society as one of double jeopardy. Since then, with the exception of Black lesbian feminists (e.g., Lorde, 1984; Parker & Jones, 1999; Smith, 1983), few psychologists have examined the experiences of Black lesbians. Notable exceptions are Greene (e.g., 1994; Greene, 1995, 1996, 1997, 1998, 2000) who has written prolifically about the "triple jeopardy" that lesbians of color experience, and Mays and Cochran (1988; Mays, Cochran, & Rhue, 1993; Peplau, Cochran, & Mays, 1997), who have researched intimate relationships among Black lesbians. Others have explored the challenges that Black lesbians, gays, and bisexuals (LGBs) experience in terms of racism within predominantly White LGB communities; heterosexism in mainstream and Black communities; and integrating their racial and sexual identities (e.g., Battle, Cohen, Warren, Fergerson, & Audam, 2002; Gutierrez, 1992; Icard, 1986; Icard, Longres, & Williams, 1996; Loiacano, 1989; Manalansan, 1996; Paradis, 1997; Stepakoff & Bowleg, 1998).

Conceptually similar to the notion of jeopardy is the notion of minority stress. Minority stress is the consequence of "stressful stimuli such as prejudice, discrimination and attendant hostility from the social environment" (Moritsugu & Sue, 1983, p. 164) on the basis of one's social status. The impact of race-related stress has been well documented in the social science and public health literature (e.g., Clark, Anderson, Clark, & Williams, 1999); and a burgeoning literature now exists on the stress relevant to other minority statuses such as sex (e.g., Klonoff & Landrine, 1995), and sexual orientation (e.g., DiPlacido, 1998; Meyer, 1995; Otis & Skinner, 1996). There exists, however, a paucity of theory or research about people such as Black lesbians who are multiply marginalized by virtue of their race,[2] sex, *and* sexual orientation. Or, as Allison (1998) has opined, "... empirical work has not yet evolved to the point of fully appreciating the stress experiences of a Jewish, African American, lesbian with a visual impairment" (p. 164). To address this gap, we designed this qualitative study to explore the experience of multiple minority stress among Black lesbians.

Beyond "triple jeopardy," however, lies another reality about which little theory or research exists; namely, that people with multiply marginalized statuses may demonstrate resilience despite minority stress (Greene, 1995; Stepakoff & Bowleg, 1998). Although definitions and measurement of resilience vary considerably, most researchers agree that two elements are essential to resilience: (1) the presence of significant stressors or challenges, and (2) positive outcomes (Kumpfer, 1999). For this study, we used Masten, Best and Garmezy's (1990) definition of resilience as "a process, capacity or outcome of successful adaptation despite challenges or threatening circumstances" (p. 426). Although a handful of resilience studies have focused on predominantly White LGB populations (e.g., Gregory, 1999), and low-income Black (presumably heterosexual) women (e.g., Todd & Worell, 2000), our literature search found no resilience studies focused on Black lesbians. Yet, research on groups such as Black lesbians may yield valuable information about how members of multiply stigmatized groups develop resilience despite multiple minority stress. Greene (1994), for example, has theorized that although managing multiple marginalized identities may increase stress, racial and ethnic minority LGBs may harbor unique resources and resiliencies honed from earlier experiences with oppression. Faced with lifetime experiences of racism and sexism, Black lesbians might be able to summon preexisting resiliency processes to cope successfully with multiple minority stressors.

THEORETICAL FRAMEWORK

The multicultural model of stress (Slavin et al., 1991) provides a useful theoretical framework for examining the multiple minority stress of Black lesbians. Of particular relevance is the model's attention to Black people's "mundane extreme environmental stress experiences" (MEES) (Allison, 1998; Peters & Massey, 1983) whereby "racism and subtle oppression are ubiquitous, constant, continuing, and mundane as opposed to an occasional misfortune" (Pierce, 1975, p. 195). Advocating for a more multiculturally inclusive conceptualization of MEES, Root's (1992) theoretically similar concept of *insidious trauma* describes the lifelong "trauma usually associated with [social statuses such as gender, color, sexual orientation, and physical ability] that are [not] valued by those in power" (p. 240).

Kumpfer's (1999) transactional model of resilience provides the theoretical framework for our focus on resilience. Her dynamic model specifies six predictors of resilience. First, stressors or challenges, such as those posed by racism, sexism, and/or heterosexism activate the resilience process. Second, external environmental contextual factors such as family, friends, and community interact to "buffer or exacerbate negative impact" (p. 189). Third, person-environment interactional processes include the use of strategies to create protective environments. Fourth are internal psychological resiliency factors such as spirituality and belief in one's uniqueness, self-esteem, problem-solving skills, and happiness (versus depression), optimism, and humor. Fifth, resiliency factors focus on stress and coping processes "learned . . . through gradual exposure to increasing challenges and stressors . . . [that] help the individual to bounce back with resilient reintegration" (p. 184). Finally, positive life outcomes predict resilient reintegration (i.e., the ability to return to a higher state of resiliency and strength) following stress. Resilience is a multidimensional construct (Kumpfer, 1999) from which a variety of positive outcomes may stem (e.g., good mental and physical health; rewarding employment, etc.). For purposes of our study, however, we chose to focus on one positive outcome: emotional social support from partners, friends, family, or other members of one's community (Barrera, 1986).

PURPOSE OF THE STUDY

At the core of qualitative research is the quest to understand "how social experience is created and given meaning" (Denzin & Lincoln, 2000, p. 8). Consequently, we chose to use qualitative methods because they are ideally suited to our goal of understanding the context of the lives of women who face challenges by virtue of their race, sex, and sexual identity. Specifically, we wanted to understand the relationship between Black lesbians' experiences of stress due to racism, sexism, and/or heterosexism, and their resiliency in spite of these stressors. First, we examined how one's status as a Black lesbian influenced the nature and frequency of single and multiple minority (i.e., racism, sexism, and/or heterosexism) stressful life experiences (Slavin et al., 1991).

Based on the MEES literature (Allison, 1998; Peters & Massey, 1983), we hypothesized that participants would cite racism and intersections of race with their other identities as the most omnipresent and challenging stressor. We reasoned that this would be the case because Black women are members of visible racial and ethnic groups (Cook & Helms, 1988) who historically have been the targets of racial oppression and discrimination in the U.S. For Black people, their visible minority status serves as a "label of primary potency . . . that deafens us to all finer discriminations that we might otherwise perceive" (Allport, 1954, p. 179). Thus, we expected that our participants' experiences of racism would be a significant stressor. Our expectation that racism would be a major and mundane stressor among participants was consistent with theory and research documenting the pervasive and deleterious effects of race-related stress for African Americans (e.g., Clark et al., 1999; Essed, 1991; Harrell, 2000; Jackson et al., 1996; Thompson, 1996).

We premised our expectations that sexism, intertwined with racism, would be a stressor on Klonoff and Landrine's (1995) findings that women of color experienced more sexist degradation than White women. We based our expectation of heterosexism as a stressor on empirical research conducted with predominantly White samples of LGBs (Brooks, 1981; DiPlacido, 1998; Meyer, 1995). As with sexism, we anticipated that experiences of heterosexist-related stress would be inseparable from racism-related stress. Finally, we anticipated that participants would report ambiguous stress fostered by the uncertainty of knowing whether they were the targets of racism, sexism, and/or heterosexism. Second, we examined the predictors of resiliency provided in the transaction model of resiliency (Kumpfer, 1999). Consistent with Greene's (1994) hypothesis that lesbians of color may be resilient because of their earlier experiences with racial and/or sexist oppression, we anticipated that the Black lesbians in our study would be resilient as operationalized in the transaction model of resiliency (Kumpfer, 1999).

METHOD

Participants and Procedures

Participants were 19 women, a subsample[3] of respondents ($N = 94$) to an anonymous questionnaire about the experiences of Black lesbians. All were attendants at a Black lesbian retreat in southern California. Signs posted around the retreat site invited prospective participants to complete the questionnaire.

To be eligible to participate in the study, respondents had to be Black/African American; identify as gay, lesbian, bisexual or queer; and be at least 18 years old. At the end of the questionnaire, respondents found a tear-off sheet inviting them to participate in a confidential interview to provide a more in-depth understanding of the experiences of Black lesbians.

Interviewees ranged in age from 26 and 68 ($M = 45$, $SD = 10.58$). The sample was predominantly African American (89.5%, $n = 17$), one woman was West Indian, and one was biracial (i.e., Black-Indian). The sample was highly educated with 42% and 26.3% reporting graduate and college degrees, respectively. Personal annual incomes ranged from less than $5,000 to between $80,00 and $89,999 (*M* = $40,000 to $49,999). Most of the respondents (68.4%) identified as lesbian, 15.8% identified as gay, 10.5% identified as other, and one woman identified as queer. Most participants were in same-sex committed relationships (57.9%); 36.8% were single, not dating; and one woman was dating. More than half of the sample (52.6%) reported a previous heterosexual marriage and 36.8% had children.

Measures

A semi-structured interview guide allowed interviewees to respond freely to six questions designed to elicit rich descriptions about the experiences of Black lesbians. The first author conducted all interviews, which were audio taped and ranged from 30 to 45 minutes. Three questions related to multiple minority stress and resilience: (1) What do you like most and least about being a Black lesbian? (2) What are some of the day-to-day challenges that you face in terms of your race, gender and/or sexual orientation? and (3) Tell me about the types of social support that you have. Do you have support for all of your identities? Prior to the interview, respondents completed a questionnaire that included demographic questions and an identification number to link interview responses. The questionnaire also included scales designed to measure self-esteem, psychosocial competence, social support, degrees of outness, and attitudes towards the mainstream LGB community, Black communities, and feminist communities.

Analyses

Audiotaped interview data were transcribed verbatim and edited to remove identifiers. We then read all of the transcripts thoroughly at least twice to become acquainted with the data. Next, we imported the data into NVivo, a qualitative management and analysis software package. We analyzed the qualitative data via three techniques derived from grounded theory: coding, memo writing, and the constant comparative method (Glaser & Strauss, 1967). Our coding phase of the analysis, progressed in three stages: open, axial and selective coding (Strauss & Corbin, 1990). During the open coding phase, we broadly coded all passages of text relevant to the experience of stress. In the axial coding phase, we refined all of the "experience of stress" codes into more distinct codes (e.g., racism-related stress; sexism-related stress). During the selective coding phase, we further refined the codes to reflect specific dimensions of the experience of, for example, heterosexism-related stress (e.g., heterosexism in Black communities). The first author conducted all phases of coding, while two coauthors independently coded for experiences of sexism and heterosexism.

At the end of the coding process, we consulted with each other to confirm that we were accurately interpreting the information that the participants provided. Analyses of the comparison of codes determined that we had arrived at the same or similar codes for the study's major themes and subcategories. For the memo writing analysis, each coder began memo writing at the initial reading of the transcripts and consistently created memos during all subsequent phases of analyses to highlight key questions about relationships in the data, to refine categories, and to ensure a close association between participants' responses and the study's research questions. In the constant comparison method stage of the analyses, we systematically compared incidents, participants or categories for similarities and differences (Glaser, 1992).

Trustworthiness of analyses. Qualitative theorists have proposed several criteria for judging the quality, or trustworthiness, of qualitative analyses (Lincoln & Guba, 1985; Miles & Huberman, 1994). We assessed the quality of our analyses via three criteria: credibility, transferability, and confirmability (Lincoln & Guba, 1985). First, we assessed whether our findings were credible by examining codes that supported key themes in the data as well as exceptions (i.e., negative case analysis). The goal of transferability is to assess whether the conclusions drawn from a qualitative study can be compared with other samples or theories. We have provided "thick description" (Lincoln & Guba, 1985, p. 316) to assist others interested in assessing the transferability of our findings. Thick descriptions include, but are not limited to, detailed accounts of the sample and discussion of prior theory. Finally, confirmability refers to the extent to which the study's methods, procedures, process of data collection and analyses, and conclusions have been described thoroughly. We have provided in the results section quotes from participants to support the conclusions that we have drawn. With the exception of some minor edits to improve clarity, all quotes are provided verbatim.

RESULTS

Minority and Multiple Minority Stress

Racism. As we anticipated, most (79%, $n = 15$)[4] of the participants cited racism as their most mundane and stressful challenge. Although two interviewees recounted personal experience with blatant racism such as being the target of racial epithets, generally, participants' discussions of their experiences of racism as a stressor focused on two themes. First, 53% ($n = 10$) of interviewees discussed their MEES experiences with racial prejudice or discrimination, such as being followed around stores or working in environments where covert racism was prevalent. Leslie,[5] a 48-year-old attorney, explained her mundane experiences with racism:

> Because it's like every day you get up and you don't know if you will get to work without one of these mad dog police pulling you over and getting into a beef and you get arrested; then you lose your job. You don't know if you'll get home at night. You don't know if when you go shopping they'll put security on you and be following you around the store.

Second, seven respondents (37%) discussed the stress of being a numerical minority in their workplaces or communities. Anita, a 43-year-old financial planner, explained, "I live in a community that is mostly White, so that's a challenge in itself."

Women's appraisal of racism as a stressor varied markedly. Although 79% ($n = 15$) of participants discussed it as a stressor, four women made no mention of racism in their interviews. Six women (32%) discussed the experience of daily encounters with racism as an annoyance. For instance, Tanisha, a 37-year-old computer technician, described the experience of being followed around stores as "a little tiresome." Only one woman, however, described mundane racism as significantly stressful. Leslie evokes the traumatic nature of this stress:

> I'm very serious when I say I feel like I am held captive here [in the U.S.]. And I am in a constant state of siege. I don't know if all Black people feel like that, but I am aware of the forces that are out here, and I am aware that they are strongly arrayed against my survival. So, as far being Black and being oppressed is concerned, I basically feel like I'm in a state of siege on a constant basis, and that I'm fighting for my life.

Sexism. Consistent with previous findings documenting the frequency with which women of color experience sexism (Klonoff & Landrine, 1995), seven

(37%) women discussed experiences with sexist degradation such as having salespeople assume that they were incompetent at home or with car repair, or being the target of sexist remarks on the street or in the workplace. Two women discussed instances of workplace sex discrimination such as pay inequity or being denied opportunities to advance professionally because they were women. Women who discussed experiences with sexism typically described it as an irritant or annoyance, compared to the more emotionally laden language that they used to discuss their experiences of racism-related stress. Presumably, this was the case because they were able to confront and oppose the sexist degradation primarily because as 37% (n = 7) noted, they felt liberated from traditional gender role norms. Thus, it is plausible that this confrontation may have attenuated the negative effects of the degradation.

Race and sex are inextricably linked social identities for Black women, however. As such, women rarely spoke about the stress of sexism absent the challenges of racism. When recounting the challenges of being Black and women, racism often emerged as a central theme, as Bernice, a 50-year-old director of a nonprofit organization, illustrates:

> I don't really experience difficulties as a woman. I mean that I don't perceive that I do. I've been able to accomplish what I wanted to from my career. I was not hindered by being a woman. Initially it was because of being Black. I had some difficulties getting into school; but, not by virtue of being a woman.

Bernice's narrative suggests that because the workplace may provide more challenges for Black lesbians as Black professionals than it does for them as women, they may attend more to racism than sexism.

Heterosexism. Participants recounted a variety of challenges with blatant heterosexism, such as being disowned by family members (10%, n = 2), being fired because of sexual orientation (n = 1), and being ostracized by a religious community (n = 1). Interviewees also described more subtle heterosexist experiences, such as not feeling comfortable about being out in the workplace (32%, n = 6); confronting heterosexist attitudes and stereotypes (32%, n = 6); having men, particularly Black men, presume that interviewees were heterosexual (26%, n = 5); and not feeling safe to engage in public displays of affection with partners (21%, n = 4). Six women (32%) reported that they experienced challenges related to self-monitoring. Specifically, participants who were not out to their families, friends or co-workers (37%, n = 7) reported considerable stress about the self-monitoring and self-silencing that they endured when discussions of social activities or relationships arose. Three interviewees (16%) were especially critical about heterosexism in Black communities, where, as Sylvia, a 39-year-old paralegal, explained, "homophobic kinds of mentalities are very rampant. . . . and being gay is like an affront to your Blackness." Yet, while these interviewees said that they perceived heterosexism in Black communities as an important challenge, none appraised it as significantly stressful. We believe that the issue here is not that Black lesbians are immune from the stress of heterosexism, but rather that despite the heterosexism in predominantly heterosexual Black communities, they rely on and wish to maintain bonds with Black communities because they buffer the stressful effects of racism.

As with sexism, interviewees' experiences of heterosexism were often intertwined with their experiences as Black women (84%, n = 16). Makeba, a 30-year-old medical clerk, shared, "I just feel like it's very difficult living as a Black woman in this lifestyle. If I had to do it all over again . . . I would walk the walk like my [heterosexual] sister." Dorothea, a 61-year-old retired realtor, explained, "I dislike the discrimination and the judgment and the oppression that comes with [being lesbian]. And the same thing applies to being Black." Finally, Vanessa's response to the challenges of being lesbian demonstrates the intersections between racism and heterosexism:

> [being a lesbian has] never held me back from gettin' a job, which is very important [to] your economical survival. So if it hasn't stopped me from gettin' a job, then there is a nothing else. . . . But I can speak for being Black, because I do remember a situation that I had when I was in [large city on East Coast]. When I was around 21, I went to a employment agency to apply for a job, and the man said, "He don't hire niggers." So I guess if I was a lesbian, he would have really thrown me down the stairs.

Several interviewees appeared to be agile at negotiating different environments to protect themselves against heterosexism. Here too, race was interwoven with their decisions. Anita, for example, noted that because she was "already challenged as a Black woman in this White society," she chose to "not add the lesbian factor" by coming out in her workplace. While 37% (n = 7) said that they were openly out as lesbians (i.e., that they openly talked about their sexual identity with family members, heterosexual friends, and/or coworkers); 37% (n = 7) said that their family members, heterosexual friends, or coworkers knew that they were lesbian, but did not discuss their sexual identity with these people; and 21% (n = 4) said that their degree of outness depended on the domain (i.e., they were out to some people such as heterosexual friends, but not out to others such as family members). Only one woman said that she was not out to her family or coworkers.

Anita's aforementioned statement suggests that because sexual orientation may be an invisible minority status for several of the women in our study, they may opt to reduce the stressful effects already inherent to their lives as Black women by choosing when, where, whether, and to whom they disclose that they are lesbians. But while choosing to be selective about coming out, presumably to reduce stress, appeared to be a viable option for some of the interviewees, two women noted that Black lesbians with nontraditional gender presentations lacked this option. Vanessa, a 62-year-old home care attendant, offered, "to be a butch lesbian, which is what my girlfriend is, [means] constantly having to deal with battles with people."

Triple jeopardy: Intersections of racism, sexism, and heterosexism. For Black lesbians, race, sex and sexual identity are intricately related not only to identity, but also to the stressful experiences that inevitably accompany these identities. Patricia's description of her identity as one in which "the deck is definitely stacked against you" because one is Black, female and lesbian resonates the notion of triple jeopardy. Patricia, a 42-year-old physical therapist, worried that the challenges associated with being a Black lesbian would "erode and wear [her] down eventually." Six interviewees (32%) discussed the challenges of negotiating environments that were predominantly Black and heterosexual or predominantly White. Cynthia, a 26-year-old physical education teacher, noted the challenges of negotiating different identity communities:

> I'm always a Black lesbian woman, no matter what. But I can be among a [predominantly] Black mixture of people and something could come up and I'm expected to think of myself solely as Black. And, they could be talking about freeing somebody like Farrakhan, who I don't particularly care for, and I don't think is woman-friendly, and definitely not gay friendly.

Candace, a 31-year-old office manager, described her experience as a Black lesbian as a challenge to survive in "a world that doesn't affirm or even want your truth." She struggled, she said, "to live in the world as fully as I can, with all of my God-given gifts and abilities, completely and wholly; instead of being fragmented or having to have dichotomized selves and realities."

In response to the threat of fragmenting identities, six women (32%) said that they often resorted to self-monitoring or code-switching strategies. This was necessary, Rosalie, a 68-year-old retired schoolteacher, explained, because, "[we live in a world in which] we don't feel totally free to conduct ourselves."

Although many participants appeared to be certain about the nature of prejudice or discrimination targeting them, four respondents (21%) suggested that it was equally stressful not knowing whether their race, sex, and/or sexual identity was the catalyst. The workplace emerged as the source of much of this ambiguous stress. Leslie recounted that when she had experienced workplace discrimination, that "quite frankly, I [didn't] know whether it's because I'm Black or because I'm woman, or queer."

Resilience

External environmental context. Interviewees noted that they often sought to balance two main external environmental factors–their families and Black communities. Sometimes, these factors buffered against the stress imposed by racism, sexism, and/or heterosexism; other times, they exacerbated it. Nancy, a 44-year-old physician, provided an example of this balancing act. Recounting the experience of her brother making advanced plans for care of his children, Nancy recalls, "he didn't want [his children] with me because I'm a lesbian. . . . So you know, that was a very rude awakening for me." Other family members, however, softened the blow of this "rude awakening" by immediately supporting Nancy's decision to care for her nieces.

As for their communities, four women (21%) mentioned their desire to affiliate with Black communities despite the perceived heterosexism within them. Gail, a 42-year-old office supply saleswoman, reflected on the tendency for some Black lesbians to face "estrangement from the Black church or Black community leaders," while at the same time wanting to remain a part of the Black church family despite its heterosexism. Leslie opined that "unlike White gays and lesbians who are always talkin' about they want to build some kind of gay and lesbian Mecca somewhere" it was important for Black LGBs to maintain ties with the Black community because these communities served as a buffer against racism.

Person-environment interactional processes. Participants described using a variety of strategies to surmount challenges in their environments and construct protective environments. Many participants took active steps to redress their feelings of isolation as Black lesbians by engaging in strategies such as: (1) seeking out books and magazines written by and for Black lesbians (11%, $n = 2$); (2) using Internet and World Wide Web searches to identify resources for Black lesbians (11%, $n = 2$); and (3) traveling to Black lesbian events, often at considerable financial expense (37%, $n = 7$). Betty, a 51-year-old fundraiser who had traveled from the east coast to attend the retreat in southern California, noted, "See, I've got to travel across country to be connected with my people." Dorothea said that her "semi-desperation" to connect with other Black lesbians prompted her to seek out assistance. She remembered: "I found myself at a recent [predominantly White] political, gay and lesbian political organization [where I said], 'Look, there is a dearth of Black lesbians up here and I'm looking to fill that. Can you help me?'"

Internal self-characteristics. Interviewees articulated a variety of internal psychological factors characteristic of resilient individuals. Among them are: (1) spiritual characteristics; (2) feelings of uniqueness; (3) self-esteem; (4) behavioral and social competencies; and (5) happiness, optimism, and humor. Seven participants (32%) invoked terms such as "gift" and "blessing" to describe their lives as Black lesbians. Others focused on the uniqueness of being Black and lesbian (26%, $n = 5$). Betty reflected, "I think that the label of being a Black lesbian is unique. It's unique in the universe and I feel uniquely gifted to be able to love a woman; to love women." Discourse about the uniqueness and spirituality of identities, however, was not universal. Flo, a 47-year-old loan officer, offered, "I just happen to love women; that's it. You know, I look at myself as a person just like every other person out here, except my sexual preference is different; that's all."

Self-esteem was a recurrent theme in several interviews. Three participants (16%) perceived self-esteem to be essential to surmounting multiple minority stress. Flo explained, "I happen to think I'm a pretty damn good person . . . [and] if someone does not like me because of my color, that's their problem." Yet, maintaining self-esteem in the midst of threats to it was not always feasible as Tanisha explained: "I like me and I feel fairly good about me unless I'm attacked in some way." As for behavioral and social competencies, five women (26%) described a variety of social and problem-solving skills honed from previous problems to negotiate social and interpersonal settings. Patricia, a child sexual abuse survivor recounted, " . . . part of my survival was [being] able to stop the perpetrator. I had a sense of power, and once I gained that sense of power, I knew how to use it."

The emotional stability and management cluster refers to characteristics such as happiness (versus depression), optimism, and humor. Although two interviewees stated that they had experienced clinical depression and were in recovery from substance abuse, five participants (26%) described their contentment with what Leslie described as, "the sense of living on the margin, and the freedom that comes with it." Women did not speak about happiness in traditional terms, but rather, appeared to conceptualize happiness as freedom from restrictive gender role norms. They relished being able to live their lives on their own terms (16%, $n = 3$), and their liberation from traditional gender role and heterosexist (37%, $n = 7$) norms that dictated that women be heterosexually married. The fact that 52.6% of the sample had been married to men may explain this sense of liberation. Bernice described her contentment this way: "I enjoy being able to express myself fully. I love being in the company of other lesbians and gay men and that's just my life. And I'm happy I made this transition [to becoming a lesbian]." Most participants' sense of liberation was mostly limited to their perceived freedom from sexist and heterosexist norms, and presumably because of the potency of racism, not race. Despite this, two participants sounded celebratory themes about being Black. Dorothea, for example, noted, "the Black part [of my identity] is just a heck of a lot of fun."

Three participants demonstrated humor despite, or possibly because, of the challenges that they encountered as Black lesbians. Dorothea recounted laughingly that living in a predominantly White small county provided her with "a lot of occasions to rise to the challenges of being a lesbian and a Black person." In spite of the multiple minority stressors they faced, two participants (11%) stated that they were determined to remain optimistic. Karen, a 47-year-old cab driver, noted that after years of battling depression, she had admitted that she was lesbian. She recalled:

> It was like a whole new world opened up. And I felt alive again and I just felt like God had given me another chance at life. And I was just so happy. And you know, I have my ups and downs, but I feel like it can be a good life for me, and it is a good life for me. And I proactively do things that will make it good for me.

Resiliency processes. Respondents engaged in a variety of resiliency processes such as actively and directly confronting oppression (26%, $n = 5$); assessing their power to change situations (11%, $n = 2$); not allowing others to define reality for them (21%, $n = 4$); and choosing not to bear the burden of other people's bigotry (11%, $n = 2$). In describing her appraisal of her power when confronted with challenges, Rosalie, the 68-year-old retired schoolteacher, said that she first assessed her power, and, "if I have no power then I ignore it." She recalled her decision to ignore men who directed racist comments towards her on the golf course:

> I had another round to play, which would only mess up my golf game if I got too mad. So I just put my hand beside my ear saying, "I didn't quite hear you," and he didn't get any louder so I did it again and he didn't get any louder so I said, "I'll ignore that one." I had no power there. If there is a situation if I feel I have been mistreated and there is management and I figure they want my money I complain. If the need arises I write a letter.

Others focused on self-definition. Sylvia recalled a time when she was working at a financial firm and a White male coworker whose propositions she had rebuffed retorted, "It must be difficult being you, being Black and being here because you must know you'll never have [what most White people have]." She noted that although she was indignant at his remark, it prompted her to reflect on the importance of self-definition: "It had a profound effect on me. It didn't weaken my spirit, but it [taught me that] a better approach might be found in trying to find a way where my approach, me, my essence, works in that world."

Positive life outcome: Socially supportive relationships. In Kumpfer's (1999) model, positive life outcomes are critical to resilience because they facilitate movement to higher states of resiliency. Our findings suggest that despite the challenges of racism, sexism, and/or heterosexism, many interviewees said that they had supportive relationships that sustained them, especially during times of stress. The sources of this support included friends (58%, n = 10), intimate partners (21%, *n* = 4), and religious communities (16%, n = 3). Interviewees expressed more reserved and ambivalent opinions about their supportive relationships with their family members, however. Although 74% of interviewees (*n* = 14) reported that they felt supported by at least one family member, all except one of these women said that this support did not always encompass their identities as Black lesbians. Instead, many families appeared to adhere to what Nancy called a "don't ask, don't tell" support policy. Namely, families were for the most part available to provide emotional support contingent on a silent pact that sexual identity issues would remain as Patricia noted, "surface-wise" or invisible. An exception to this rule was Gail, who noted, "I feel that my family, supports every aspect of me. My lesbian self, my female self; my educated self . . . My healthy self, my unhealthy self. My family is there for me in every aspect."

Despite yearning for greater acceptance and support from their families, many interviewees said that they cherished the supportive relationships that they had with their friends, partners, and religious communities. Candace, aptly summarized the influence of fulfilling and supportive relationships on resilient reintegration:

> I've been blessed by having some really incredible friends. . . . And I've been blessed with a partner who accepts me absolutely and supports me, in all of my realities. . . . I don't have a lot of support [from my family or in this community], but I have some real solid pieces and it makes a difference when things are incredibly hard or you're met with silence or just simple challenges of dealing as a lesbian, a Black lesbian woman in this world.

DISCUSSION

We designed this study to explore the experiences of multiple minority stress and resilience among a sample of lesbians attending a Black lesbian retreat. We anticipated that most of the participants would discuss racism as a mundane and significant stressor, and the data supported this assumption. We also expected that participants would discuss sexism and heterosexism as stressors, particularly within the context of race and racism, and this was also the case. Specifically, participants often contextualized their experiences of sexism and heterosexism-related stress, through the prism of race and racism. Also as expected, some participants discussed the experience of ambiguous stress prompted by their uncertainty about whether a stressor was due to racism, sexism, and/or heterosexism. Thus, our findings provide empirical support for the "triple jeopardy" experience of Black lesbians that Greene (1995) has articulated. Finally, despite, or possibly in reaction to this triple jeopardy of racism, sexism, and heterosexism, we anticipated that the women in our study would be resilient, as operationalized by the six predictors of Kumpfer's (1999) transactional model of resilience. Our data supported the notion of resilience among the Black lesbians interviewed for this study.

Implications of the Study

Qualitative methods facilitate the exploration of rich contextual data about people's lives; and thus were ideal for our study. Nonetheless, several caveats about the study are warranted. First, because of our study's small sample size and the method of recruitment, our findings cannot be generalized to Black lesbians beyond those who participated in our study. Another limitation is that because our participants constituted a self-selected sample of women attending a retreat that billed itself as a "celebration of Black lesbians," they may be more inherently resilient than those not attending such a retreat, or even those who did not volunteer to be interviewed. Although research involving randomly selected samples of Black lesbians is needed, the infinitesimal size and stigmatized nature of this population makes attempts to obtain random samples arduous, though not impossible. Finally, because the women in our study were predominantly middle-class and highly educated, it is plausible that their class privilege may have influenced their frequency and appraisal of multiple minority stress. Research suggests that stress is often exacerbated among Blacks with lower socioeconomic status (SES) and that the appraisal of racism as overt or covert varies as a function of one's SES (Clark et al., 1999). Thus more research is needed to understand how factors such as SES as well as gender presentation may influence Black lesbians' experiences with overt and covert racism, sexism and/or heterosexism.

Ransford (1980) has called research on the jeopardy and advantages of multiple social identities a "veritable empirical wasteland" (p. 272). His assessment is still relevant. Despite the preponderance of theories on minority stress, virtually no research exists on the experience of multiple minority stress. Our findings suggest that more research is needed to understand not only multiple minority stress, but also how ambiguous attributions about multiple minority stressors influence the nature and severity of stress. Moreover, our study suggests that including nontraditional populations such as Black lesbians in psychological research portends a variety of new perspectives and understandings about a panoply of social psychological concepts such as the self and multiple social identity development; to name just a few.

As for resilience, the majority of published studies have been conducted with children and adolescents, and thus little is known about resilience in adults. Moreover, researchers posit stress as a necessary catalyst for resilience. Our research suggests, however, that we need to learn more about the nature of stress along multiple dimensions posed by factors such as racism, sexism and/or heterosexism, as well as stressors related to other identity statuses such as low socioeconomic or disability status. Black lesbians' intersecting identities as people who are Black, women, and lesbian also provide important implications for Black, feminist and LGB advocacy. Because of the nexus of intersecting identities (combined of course with others such as disability status and SES) organizations working for social change, if they are to be effective in their mission, must shed the illusion of the homogeneity of experience (Lorde, 1984). They must actively address within group diversity across dimensions such as race, sex, gender, sexual identity, SES and disability.

CONCLUSION

Historically, psychology has focused on pathology rather than positive mental health. Thus, while we know much about the debilitating effects of minority stress, we know little about the negative or positive effects of having a multiply stigmatized identity. In a departure from solely deficit-focused models of minority experience, we found that the Black lesbians in our study were resilient despite the multiple minority stress they experience. Of course, as we have previously acknowledged, it is also likely that the participants in our study were inherently resilient by virtue of their participation in an African American lesbian retreat. This notwithstanding, we believe that it is essential to acknowledge the ubiquitous and pernicious effects of racist, sexist, and heterosexist oppression and the institutional structures that bolster them. Our goal was not to decontextualize the experience of resilience, but rather to illustrate an affirmative dimension of the lives of a sample of Black lesbians despite racism, sexism, and/or heterosexism. Moreover, we recognize that while research on multiple minority stress and resilience among Black lesbians may be novel in psychology, Lorde (1984) reminds us that these experiences are not new to those who live on the margins of race, sex, and sexual identity:

> Those of us who stand outside the circle of this society's definition of acceptable women; those of us who have been forged in the crucibles of difference–those of us who are poor, who are lesbians, who are Black, who are older–know that *survival is not an academic* skill. . . . It is learning how to take our differences and make them strengths. (p. 112)

NOTES

1. We use the term *Black* to describe the sociopolitical experiences of people of African descent who reside in the U.S. regardless of ethnicity (e.g., Latina, African American, Caribbean).

2. Historically, social scientists have used the term *race* to denote phenotypic characteristics such as skin color or hair texture. The term is at best quasi-biological, however, because one's phenotype "reveals virtually nothing about [one's] genotype" (Helms, 1994, p. 297). In this article, we use the term *race* to denote the collective sociopolitical history of racial oppression that African Americans, in particular, and Blacks, in general, have experienced in the U.S.

3. We statistically compared the subsample of women who volunteered to be interviewed to the questionnaire-only sample ($n = 75$) on several outcomes of interest (i.e., degree of outness, social support, self-esteem, and psychosocial competence), as well as a number of demographic variables. We found no statistical differences between the two groups on any outcome measure. Our analyses of demographic differences found that interviewees were older ($M = 43$ years vs. 36 years) and more educated (mean *of* some graduate school vs. some college degree) than the questionnaire-only sample. We found no differences in income or location of residence (i.e., rural, suburban, urban). Data from all of the interviewees are included in the results.

4. Rather than relying on ambiguous descriptors such as "some" or "most," we indicate percentages and numbers to precisely represent the data. We derived these percentages and numbers from the codes related to interviewee's transcripts. Specifically, we assessed the degree to which an experience was stressful based on whether the interviewee mentioned it and our analysis of the quality of the stress (i.e., whether the interviewee discussed it as a major stressor versus, for example, an irritation or annoyance).

5. To protect confidentiality, all names and occupations have been changed.

REFERENCES

Allison, K. W. (1998). Stress and oppressed social category membership. In C. Stangor (Ed.), *Prejudice: The target's perspective* (pp. 145-170). San Diego, CA: Academic Press.

Allport, G. W. (1954). *The nature of prejudice.* Cambridge, MA: Addison-Wesley.

Barrera, M. (1986). Distinctions between social support concepts, measures, and models. *American Journal of Community Psychology, 14*(4), 413-445.

Battle, J., Cohen, C. J., Warren, D., Fergerson, G., & Audam, S. (2002). *Say it loud: I'm Black and I'm Proud: Black Pride Survey 2000.* New York: The Policy Institute of the National Gay and Lesbian Task Force.

Beale, F. (1970). Double jeopardy: To be black and female. In T. Cade (Ed.), *The Black woman* (pp. 90-100). New York: Signet.

Brooks, V. R. (1981). *Minority stress and lesbian women.* Lexington, MA: Lexington Books.

Clark, R., Anderson, N. B., Clark, V. R., & Williams, D. R. (1999). Racism as a stressor for African Americans: A biopsychosocial model. *American Psychologist, 54*(10), 805-816.

Cook, D. A., & Helms, J. E. (1988). Visible racial/ethnic group supervisees' satisfaction with cross-cultural supervision as predicted by relationship characteristics. *Journal of Counseling Psychology, 35*(3), 268-274.

Denzin, N. K., & Lincoln, Y. S. (2000). Introduction: The discipline and practice of qualitative research. In Y. S. Lincoln (Ed.), *Handbook of qualitative research* (2nd ed., pp. 1-28). Thousand Oaks, CA: Sage.

DiPlacido, J. (1998). Minority stress among lesbians, gay men, and bisexuals: A consequence of heterosexism, homophobia, and stigmatization. In G. M. Herek (Ed.), *Stigma and sexual orientation: Understanding prejudice against lesbians, gay men, and bisexuals* (pp. 138-159). Thousand Oaks, CA: Sage, Inc.

Essed, P. (1991). *Understanding everyday racism: An interdisciplinary theory.* Newbury Park, CA: Sage.

Glaser, B. G. (1992). *Basics of grounded theory analysis: Emergence vs. forcing.* Mill Valley, CA: Sociology Press.

Glaser, B. G., & Strauss, A. (1967). *The discovery of grounded theory: Strategies for qualitative research.* Chicago: Aldine.

Greene, B. (1994). Ethnic-minority lesbians and gay men: Mental health and treatment issues. *Journal of Consulting and Clinical Psychology, 62*(2), 243-251.

Greene, B. (1995). Lesbian women of color: Triple jeopardy. In B. Greene (Ed.), *Women of color: Integrating ethnic and gender identities in psychotherapy* (pp. 389-427). New York: Guilford Publications.

Greene, B. (1996). Lesbians and gay men of color: The legacy of ethnosexual mythologies in heterosexism. In E. R. L. Bond (Ed.), *Preventing heterosexism and homophobia.* Sage.

Greene, B. (Ed.) (1997). *Ethnic and cultural diversity among lesbians and gay men.* Thousand Oaks, CA: Sage.

Greene, B. (1998). Family, ethnic identity, and sexual orientation: African-American lesbians and gay men. In C. J. Patterson & A. R. D'Augelli (Eds.), *Lesbian, gay, and bisexual identities in families: Psychological perspectives* (pp. 40-52). New York: Oxford University Press.

Greene, B. (2000). African American lesbian and bisexual women in feminist-psychodynamic psychotherapies: Surviving and thriving between a rock and a hard place. In L. C. Jackson & B. Greene (Eds.), *Psychotherapy with African American women: Innovations in psychodynamic perspective and practice* (pp. 82-125). New York: The Guilford Press.

Gregory, C. J. (1999). *Resiliency among lesbian and bisexual women during the process of self-acceptance and disclosure of their sexual orientation.* Unpublished doctoral dissertation, University of Rhode Island.

Gutierrez, F. J. D. S. H. (1992). Gay, lesbian, and African American: Managing the integration of identities. In F. J. G. S. H. Dworkin (Ed.), *Counseling gay men and lesbians* (pp. 141-156). Alexandria, VA: American Association of Counseling and Development.

Harrell, S. P. (2000). A multidimensional conceptualization of racism-related stress: Implications for the well-being of people of color. *American Journal of Orthopsychiatry, 70*(1), 42-57.

Helms, J. E. (1994). The conceptualization of racial identity and other "racial" constructs. In E. J. Trickett & R. J. Watts (Eds.), *Human diversity: Perspectives on people in context. The Jossey Bass social and behavioral science series* (pp. 285-311). San Francisco, CA: Jossey-Bass.

Icard, L. (1986). Black gay men and conflicting social identities: Sexual orientation versus racial identity. *Journal of Social Work and Human Sexuality, 4*(1-2), 83-93.

Icard, L. D., Longres, J. F., & Williams, J. H. (1996). An applied research agenda for homosexually active men of color. *Journal of Gay and Lesbian Social Services, 5*(2-3), 139-164.

Jackson, J. S., Brown, T. N., Williams, D. R., Torres, M., Sellers, S. L., & Brown, K. (1996). Racism and the physical and mental health status of African Americans: A thirteen year national panel study. *Ethnicity and Disease, 6*(1-2), 132-147.

Klonoff, E. A., & Landrine, H. (1995). The Schedule of Sexist Events: A measure of lifetime and recent sexist discrimination in women's lives. *Psychology of Women Quarterly, 19*(4), 439-472.

Kumpfer, K. L. (1999). Factors and processes contributing to resilience: The resilience framework. In M. D. Glantz & J. L. Johnson (Eds.), *Resilience and development: Positive life adaptations* (pp. 179-224). New York: Kluwer Academic/Plenum Publishers.

Lincoln, Y. S., & Guba, E. G. (1985). *Naturalistic inquiry*. Beverly Hills, CA: Sage.

Loiacano, D. K. (1989). Gay identity issues among Black Americans: Racism, homophobia, and the need for validation. *Journal of Counseling and Development, 68*(1), 21-25.

Lorde, A. (1984). *Sister outsider: Essays and speeches*. Trumansburg, NY: Crossing Press.

Manalansan, M. F. I. V. (1996). Double minorities: Latino, Black, and Asian men who have sex with men. In K. M. Cohen (Ed.), *The lives of lesbians, gays, and bisexuals: Children to adults* (pp. 393-415). Orlando, FL, US: Harcourt Brace College Publishers.

Masten, A. S., Best, K. M., & Garmezy, N. (1990). Resilience and development: Contributions from the study of children who overcome adversity. *Development and Psychopathology*, *2*(4), 425-444.

Mays, V. M., & Cochran, S. D. (1988). The Black women's relationship project: A national survey of Black lesbians. In W. Scott (Ed.), *The sourcebook on lesbian/gay health care* (2 ed., pp. 54-62). Washington, DC: The National Lesbian/Gay Health Foundation.

Mays, V. M., Cochran, S. D., & Rhue, S. (1993). The impact of perceived discrimination on the intimate relationships of Black lesbians. *Journal of Homosexuality*, *25*(4), 1-14.

Meyer, I. H. (1995). Minority stress and mental health in gay men. *Journal of Health and Social Behavior*, *36*(March), 38-56.

Miles, M. B., & Huberman, A. M. (1994). *Qualitative data analysis: An expanded sourcebook* (2nd ed.). Thousand Oaks, CA: Sage.

Moritsugu, J., & Sue, S. (1983). Minority status as a stressor. In R. D. Felner (Ed.), *Preventive psychology: Theory, research and practice* (pp. 162-174). New York: Pergammon.

Otis, M. D., & Skinner, W. F. (1996). The prevalence of victimization and its effect on mental well-being among lesbian and gay people. *Journal of Homosexuality*, *30*(3), 93-117.

Paradis, B. A. (1997). Multicultural identity and gay men in the era of AIDS. *American Journal of Orthopsychiatry*, *67*(2), 300 307.

Parker, M. N., & Jones, R. T. (1999). Minority status stress: Effect on the psychological and academic functioning of African-American students. *Journal of Gender, Culture, and Health*, *4*(1), 61-82.

Peplau, L. A., Cochran, S. D., & Mays, V. M. (1997). A national survey of the intimate relationships of African American lesbians and gay men: A look at commitment, satisfaction, sexual behavior, and HIV disease. In B. Greene (Ed.), *Ethnic and cultural diversity among lesbians and gay men* (pp. 11-38). Thousand Oaks, CA: Sage.

Peters, M. F., & Massey, G. (1983). Mundane extreme environmental stress in family stress theories: The case of Black families in White America. *Marriage and Family Review*, *6*(1-2), 193-218.

Pierce, C. (1975). The mundane extreme environment and its effects on learning. In S. G. Brainard (Ed.), *Learning disabilities: Issues and recommendations for research.* Washington, DC: National Institute of Education.

Ransford, H. E. (1980). The prediction of social behavior and attitudes. In H. Ransford (Ed.), *Social stratification: A multiple hierarchy approach* (pp. 265-295). Boston: Allyn & Bacon.

Root, M. P. (1992). Reconstructing the impact of trauma on personality. In M. Ballou (Ed.), *Personality and psychopathology: Feminist reappraisals* (pp. 229-266). NY: Guilford.

Slavin, L. A., Rainer, K. L., McCreary, M. L., & Gowda, K. K. (1991). Toward a multicultural model of the stress process. *Journal of Counseling and Development*, *70*, 156-163.

Smith, B. (Ed.) (1983). *Home girls: A Black feminist anthology*. New York: Kitchen Table: Women of Color Press.

Stepakoff, S., & Bowleg, L. (1998). Sexual identity in sociocultural context: Clinical implications of multiple marginalizations. In W. G. Herron (Ed.), *Mental health, mental illness and personality development in a diverse society: A source book* (pp. 618-653). Northvale, NJ: Jason Aronson, Inc.

Strauss, A., & Corbin, J. (1990). *Basics of qualitative research.* London: Sage.

Thompson, V. L. (1996). Perceived experiences of racism as stressful life events. *Community Mental Health Journal, 32*(3), 223-233.

Todd, J. L., & Worell, J. (2000). Resilience in low-income, employed, African American women. *Psychology of Women Quarterly, 24*(2), 119-128.

Cast into the Wilderness: The Impact of Institutionalized Religion on Lesbians

Deana F. Morrow

SUMMARY. This article addresses the impact of traditional Judeo-Christian religion as a tool of social injustice against lesbians. The prejudices of sexism and heterosexism in religion are addressed. Biblical interpretations of woman-to-woman sexuality are reviewed. Primary Judeo-Christian groups, and their respective positions on homosexuality, are identified. Conversion therapy as a weapon of oppression against lesbians is addressed. Mechanisms for religious/spiritual transformation and empowerment are discussed, and suggestions for therapeutic intervention with lesbians recovering from religious trauma are offered.

Deana F. Morrow, PhD, LPC, LCSW, ACSW, is Associate Professor and BSW Program Director in the Department of Social Work at the University of North Carolina at Charlotte, where she teaches courses in clinical social work practice, including practice with gay, lesbian, bisexual, and transgender persons. She is a Licensed Professional Counselor and Licensed Clinical Social Worker with a clinical practice background in the areas of mental health, health care, and aging.

Address correspondence to: Deana F. Morrow, The University of North Carolina at Charlotte, Department of Social Work, 9201 University City Boulevard, Charlotte, NC 28223 (E-mail: dmorrow@uncc.edu).

[Haworth co-indexing entry note]: "Cast into the Wilderness: The Impact of Institutionalized Religion on Lesbians." Morrow, Deana F. Co-published simultaneously in *Journal of Lesbian Studies* (Harrington Park Press, an imprint of The Haworth Press, Inc.) Vol. 7, No. 4, 2003, pp. 109-123; and: *Trauma, Stress, and Resilience Among Sexual Minority Women: Rising Like the Phoenix* (ed: Kimberly F. Balsam) Harrington Park Press, an imprint of The Haworth Press, Inc., 2003, pp. 109-123. Single or multiple copies of this article are available for a fee from The Haworth Document Delivery Service [1-800-HAWORTH, 9:00 a.m. - 5:00 p.m. (EST). E-mail address: docdelivery@haworthpress.com].

http://www.haworthpress.com/store/product.asp?sku=J155

10.1300/J155v07n04_08

KEYWORDS. Lesbian, gay, religion, spirituality, heterosexism, trauma

Institutionalized religious doctrines are a major source of social oppression for many lesbians. Some theologians have asserted that social injustice based on sexual orientation is a sin for which many mainstream religions have yet to repent (Gomes, 1996; Heward, 1989; Spong, 1988, 1991, 1998). This article will address the impact of Judeo-Christian religion as a mechanism of control over lesbian sexuality. The prejudices of sexism and heterosexism in religion will be addressed, and interpretations of Biblical passages relative to lesbian sexuality will be examined. Avenues for personal transformation and empowerment toward an ethic of religious social justice will be reviewed, and implications for therapeutic work with lesbian clients traumatized by religious oppression will be offered.

RELIGION AS A SOCIAL INSTITUTION

A social institution may be defined as a system of social relationships and cultural elements that represent standardized, authorized mechanisms for structuring behavior and social expectations among people (Appleby & Anastas, 1998). Examples of social institutions include the family, business, government, politics, and education (Popple & Leighninger, 2002). Organized religion is among the most powerful and influential social institutions in the United States. In many instances, religious doctrines shape the principles around which people define and construct the very essence of morality in their lives. As a social institution, religion contributes significantly to broad moral constructs, not the least of which are gender and sexuality.

SEXISM IN RELIGION

The role of sexism in Judeo-Christian religion is rooted in the patriarchal cultural context of Biblical writings in which women were viewed as subordinate to–even as the property of–men. Religion-based sexism continues to be manifested through the perpetuation of a "power-over" (Heyward, 1989) patriarchy maintained by mostly male religious leaders, many of whom continue to define the roles of women and men based on a literal interpretation of scripture that was written over 2000 years ago.

The concept of deity itself is described in Judeo-Christian tradition as a male-centered image that is referred to as "God the Father" (Spong, 1998). As maleness has been constructed to define the presence of God, so too has it assumed a superior status in the construction of primary social institutions, including religion, families, business, politics, and communities. Thus, even though the Judeo-Christian tradition came into existence in a world radically different from the current world (Spong, 1998), its impact in perpetuating a sexist cultural climate continues. As a result, women's voices are too often marginalized in leadership and decision-making roles in communities of faith and in the very family structures that are so often defined by the male decision-makers of those faith communities. Furthermore, compared to men, women continue to encounter higher rates of poverty and fewer professional options, and they earn lower salaries for work that is comparable to their male counterparts (Akabas, 1995; Faludi 1991).

HETEROSEXISM IN RELIGION

A woman who intimately loves another woman is considered particularly vile in traditional Judeo-Christian teachings. Institutional religion has long been a mechanism for heterosexist intolerance and oppression of those who are same-sex identified in their intimate lives (Clark, Brown, & Hochstein, 1989; Davidson, 2000; Hilton, 1992; McNeill, 1993; Spong, 1991, 1998). Heterosexism is defined as the belief in the superiority of a heterosexual orientation over other forms of sexual orientation (Morrow, 1996). Even though the moral development of gays and lesbians has been found to be equivalent to, or in some cases beyond that of comparable heterosexual samples (Bordisso, 1988; Mitchell, 1983; Thompson, 1991), mainstream religion continues to define gays and lesbians as immoral and spiritually corrupt. It is no wonder then that lesbians would be hostile toward a Judeo-Christian ethic that devalues the very essence of who they are, the intimate relationships that encircle their lives, and their capacity for religious experience.

Research on both church-involved and non-church-involved lesbians suggests that they tend to experience conflict between their sexual orientation and their religious beliefs (Mahaffy, 1996). In a study of 66 lesbians and gay men, Shuck and Liddle (2001) identified the sources of such conflict as gay-negative religious teachings and scriptural interpretations, guilt and shame created by religious doctrine, gay-negative church atmospheres, and a fear of feeling exposed as a gay or lesbian person in nonaffirming religious settings. Participants in the Shuck and Liddle study coped with their dissonance in a number of ways. Some came to reject organized religion entirely. Others maintained their personal spiritual practices even though they stopped attending religious services. And still others reported shifting from oppressive Judeo-Christian religions to traditions that were more gay and lesbian welcoming and inclusive (e.g., Metropolitan Community Church, United Church of Christ, Unity, and Unitarian Universalist).

In another study, Rodriquez and Ouellette (2000) investigated the extent to which lesbian and gay Christians in a gay-affirmative church had integrated their sexual orientation identity with their religious identity. Despite their involvement in a gay-affirmative religious setting, 25% of the study participants had not fully integrated their sexual orientation identity with their religious identity. Perhaps this finding is indicative of the depth of woundedness, shame and guilt engendered by lifelong social and religious heterosexism. Interestingly, lesbians in the study were more likely than gay men to be fully integrated (88% versus 64%). This gender difference may reflect, in part, other research that identifies women as having a stronger personal faith, a deeper commitment to religious beliefs, and a higher level of involvement in worship services than men (Thompson, 1991).

Rodriquez and Ouellette (2000) propose four options which lesbians and gays may engage when coping with internal conflict created by religious heterosexism. The first option is to reject their religious identity. Over 60% of lesbians and gay men report that religion is no longer an important part of their lives (Singer & Deschamps, 1994). The second option is to reject their lesbian or gay identity. In such cases, people may seek to "pray away" their same-sex identification, suppress their sexual orientation identity, or seek out religiously-based forms of conversion therapy in order to try to "change" their sexual orientation to heterosexual.

The third option is compartmentalization, which is keeping one's sexual orientation identity separate from one's religious identity. This option is reflected in the Cass Model (Cass, 1979, 1984a, 1984b) of gay and lesbian identity development as the stage of Tolerance where people tend to compartmentalize their lives into, on the one hand, adopting an openly lesbian or gay identity among accepting friends while, on the other hand, maintaining a presumed heterosexual identity among others who might be less accepting. The Cass Model is a six stage model that depicts gay and lesbian identity development as moving through a series of sequential stages in which individuals progress from less to more self-accepting as gay or lesbian and from less to more open in disclosing their sexual identity as one component of their overall personal identity.

The last option according to Rodriguez and Ouellette (2000) is identity integration. With this option there is an integration of both a lesbian or gay identity and a religious identity. This option parallels the Synthesis stage of the Cass Model where persons have synthesized, or integrated, a same-sex identity throughout all aspects of their lives. Avenues for supporting and facilitating the integration of a lesbian identity with a religious or spiritual identity can include involvement with lesbian-affirmative religions and spiritual practices, the study of lesbian-affirming and feminist theologies, and involvement with lesbian supportive religious and spiritual groups.

BIBLICAL INTERPRETATIONS

Among the most severe forms of Judeo-Christian oppression toward women in general, and lesbians in particular, have been sexist and heterosexist interpretations of Biblical writings. Scriptural interpretation has been used in the past to justify slavery and racism, and it continues to be used by many today to support the subordination of women to men and the condemnation of same-sex identified people (Gomes, 1996; Heyward, 1989; Spong, 1998; Thistlewhite, 1991). Ascribing to a literal interpretation of the Bible has been identified as the major predictor of negative attitudes toward lesbians and gays (Taylor, 2000). Many theologians (Gomes, 1996; Heyward, 1989; Spong, 1998; Thistlewhite, 1991) now emphasize the importance of considering scriptural writings within the historical, cultural, and societal context in which they were written.

It is interesting to note that, while there are more than 350 Biblical admonishments pertaining to heterosexual sexuality, there are only seven passages targeted toward same sex behavior (More Light Presbyterians of Charlotte, 2001). And of those seven passages, only one verse (Romans 1:26) specifically addresses what has been interpreted as woman-to-woman sexual behavior: "For this reason God gave them up to degrading passions. Their women exchanged natural intercourse for unnatural . . . " (Holy Bible, New Revised Standard Version, 1989). As further context for that passage, Verse 27 continues, "And in the same way also the men, giving up natural intercourse with women, were consumed with passion for one another. Men committed shameless acts with men and received in their own persons the due penalty for their error."

Literal interpretations of Verse 26 suggest it is clear and compelling in condemning woman-to-woman sexual behavior. Yet, in considering the historical cultural context in which it was written, it is important to recognize that a lesbian sexual orientation was not scientifically understood then as something that could be natural. Even the term, homosexuality, was not coined until the nineteenth century and does not appear in any of the original Biblical manuscripts (Gomes, 1996; McNeill, 1993). Johnson (1992) addresses the lack of scientific information available to the Biblical writers:

> We need to acknowledge that the Gospel writers and the missionary Paul did not possess the psychological, sociological, and sexological knowledge which now inform our theological reflections about human sexuality. They knew nothing of sexual orientation or of the natural heterosexual-bisexual-homosexual continuum that exists in human life. They did not postulate that persons engaging in same-gender sex acts could have been expressing their natural sexuality. (pp. 145-146)

Using the Bible to declare that women loving women is unnatural or evil is inconclusive at best. The Biblical writers did not address the concept of loving, committed lesbian relationships (Bennett, 1998). What they addressed instead had to do with exploitive behaviors and behaviors that were understood at the time to be beyond a person's "natural" inclinations (Creech, 1998). We know today that developing an intimate relationship with a woman is as natural for a lesbian as developing intimacy with a man is for a heterosexual woman, in that research strongly supports an innate biological predisposition toward sexual orientation (Bailey & Pillard, 1991; Bailey, Pillard, Neale, & Agyei, 1993; LeVay, 1991; Hamer, Hu, Magnuson, Hu, & Pattatucci, 1993).

Furthermore, the subject of homosexuality was not mentioned in the Ten Commandments nor in the Summary of the Law (Gomes, 1996). Nor was it addressed by Jesus (Bennett, 1998; Spong, 1988, 1991). Gomes (1996) provides the following compelling statement regarding the Biblical condemnation of homosexuality:

> . . . No credible case against homosexuality or homosexuals can be made from the Bible unless one chooses to read scripture in a way that simply sustains the existing prejudice against homosexuality and homosexuals. The combination of ignorance and prejudice under the guise of morality makes the religious community, and its abuse of scripture in this regard, itself morally culpable. (p. 147)

POSITIONS OF PRIMARY RELIGIOUS GROUPS

Despite compelling evidence to the contrary, many of the largest Judeo-Christian religious groups and denominations in the United States continue to define homosexuality as sinful. Religious groups that have adopted particularly anti-gay positions include the Roman Catholic Church, the Southern Baptist Convention, the Church of Jesus Christ of Latter Day Saints (Mormonism), and Orthodox Judaism (Bennett, 1998). The historically African American Christian denominations of the National Baptist Convention, the Church of God in Christ, and the African Methodist Episcopal Church have chosen to offer no official policy statements on homosexuality. Even absent official policies, however, traditional African American religious communities are described as unofficially nonaccepting of homosexuality (Bennett, 1998; Boykin, 1996).

Religious groups identified as more accepting toward lesbians and gays include the United Church of Christ, the Episcopal Church, Unity, Quaker Friends Meetings, and Unitarian Universalists, as well as various churches across denominations who, as an act of social justice, have deliberately separated themselves from heterosexist denominational doctrine. There are two major gay, lesbian, bisexual, and transgender focused Christian denominations: the Metropolitan Community Church and the Unity Fellowship Church Movement which is populated primarily by African American membership. In addition, many lesbians have pursued less mainstream forms of religious and spiritual practices that are lesbian-affirming, including Native American spirituality, feminist-based spirituality, and Wiccan practices (Roscoe, 1988; Thistlewhite, 1991).

Table 1 offers further information about major Judeo-Christian religious groups and their positions on homosexuality, their willingness to accept lesbians and gays as clergy, and their positions on holy unions (gay and lesbian commitment ceremonies).

CONVERSION THERAPY

Conversion therapy, also known as reparative therapy, is a systematic means for attempting to change a person's sexual orientation from lesbian or gay to heterosexual. Such therapy typically occurs within the context of a fundamental or conservative religious setting, and commonly includes prayer, exorcism, religious-based guilt inducement, and even punishment-oriented forms of behavior modification (Ritter & O'Neill, 1989; White, 1995). Conversion therapy is often conducted by religious followers rather than credentialed psychotherapists.

There is no empirical evidence that conversion therapy is successful in actually changing sexual orientation (Haldeman, 1994; Human Rights Campaign, 1999). Numerous mental health professional associations, including the

TABLE 1. Major Judeo-Christian Religions: Position on Homosexuality, Acceptance of Gay/Lesbian Clergy, and Endorsement of Holy Union Ceremonies*

Religion	**Position on Homosexuality**	**Acceptance of Gay/Lesbian Clergy**	**Sanctions Holy Union Ceremonies for Gay/Lesbian Couples**
Roman Catholic Church (61.2 million members, largely Caucasian)	A gay/lesbian orientation is unnatural and disordered. Gay/lesbian Catholics should remain celibate for life.	All Roman Catholic clergy must remain celibate, thus obscuring overt sexual orientation.	No
Southern Baptist Convention (15.7 million members, largely Caucasian)	Homosexuality is sinful, impure, degrading, shameful, unnatural, indecent and perverted. The SBC purports to bar any congregation that acts to affirm, approve, or endorse homosexual behavior. The SBC insists that gays/lesbians remain celibate or, more commonly, change their sexual orientation through prayer and conversion therapy.	No	No
United Methodist Church (8.5 million members, largely Caucasian)	Does not condone the practice of homosexuality and considers it incompatible with Christian teaching. Gay/lesbian sexual practices are sin.	No, if a "practicing" gay/lesbian. Yes, if remain celibate.	No
National Baptist Convention, USA, Inc. (8.2 million members, largely African American)	No official policy. Unofficially does not condone homosexuality.	Unofficially, no.	Unofficially, no.
Church of God in Christ (5.5 million members, largely African American)	No official policy. Unofficially does not condone homosexuality.	Unofficially, no.	Unofficially, no.
Evangelical Lutheran Church of America (5.2 million members, largely Caucasian)	Gays/lesbians are welcome to participate fully in the life of the congregations.	Yes, if remain celibate.	No

Religion	Position on Homosexuality	Acceptance of Gay/Lesbian Clergy	Sanctions Holy Union Ceremonies for Gay/Lesbian Couples
Church of Jesus Christ of Latter Day Saints (4-8 million members, largely Caucasian)	Homosexuality is perverse, immoral. Encourages conversion therapy. Discipline for "practicing" gays/lesbians can include probation, exclusion from sacraments, or excommunication.	No	No
Judaism (3.9 million members, largely Caucasian) 1) Orthodox Judaism	Sexual relations between same gender people are sinful.	No	No
2) Conservative Judaism	No longer considers homosexuality an abomination. Supports nondiscrimination policies for gays/lesbians in civil society.	No	No
3) Reform Judaism (the largest Jewish movement)	Homosexuality is not a sin. Advocates freedom from employment discrimination in civil society. Supports marriage rights for gays/lesbians.	Yes	Permits, but does not officially sanction, holy unions.
4) Reconstructionist Judaism	Fully supportive of gays/lesbians	Yes	Officially sanctions holy unions.
Presbyterian Church, U.S.A. (3.6 million members, largely Caucasian)	Homosexuality is sin. It is not God's wish for humanity. It is neither a state nor condition like race, but rather a result of living in a fallen world.	Only if celibate. All church leaders must be heterosexually married or celibate.	No
African Methodist Episcopal Church (3.6 million members, largely African American membership)	No official policy. Unofficially does not condone homosexuality.	Unofficially, no.	Unofficially, no.

*Information compiled from: Bennett, L. (1998). *Mixed blessings: Organized religion and gay and lesbian Americans in 1998.* Washington, D.C.: Human Rights Campaign Foundation.

American Medical Association, the American Psychological Association, the National Association of Social Workers, and the American Counseling Association, have developed policies stating the practice of conversion therapy is unethical–even harmful–to clients. Such therapeutic practices serve to reinforce internalized homophobia and societal heterosexism. Ethical therapy is centered not on seeking to change sexual orientation, but rather on helping individuals cope with the effects of internalized homophobia and cultural heterosexism.

TRANSFORMATION AND EMPOWERMENT

Religion is central to the landscape of American culture. Most Americans are reared in families that ascribe to some type of religious belief or faith tradition (Shuck & Liddle, 2001). Therefore, many lesbians are reared in a religious context. The importance of religion, spirituality, and faith traditions cannot be underestimated. People turn to their religious traditions for comfort and solace in times of trouble, and for celebration and validation in times of joy. For some, the very rhythm of their lives beats to the seasons of religious ritual and tradition. Yet, what are lesbians to do when the religions upon which they have assembled their beliefs and spiritual practices cast them aside because of their sexual orientation? Where do they turn when there is no longer a place for them at the table of faith? How do they heal from the trauma of knowing their sexual orientation is viewed as something for which they must repent and be healed?

Because of religious injustice due to their sexual orientation, many lesbians have suffered family rejection, social rejection, loss of their church homes, and loss of the faith communities in which they were reared. Indeed, the multiple losses experienced by lesbians because of religious injustice are deep and profound. While such losses are traumatic, they may also become a "springboard for religious transformation" (Ritter & O'Neill, 1989, p. 12). Critical feminist analysis of the ways in which religion is used to perpetuate heterosexism and the disempowerment of lesbian women can be a catalyst for empowerment and transformation. The reader is referred to Christ (1998), Christ and Plaskow (1992), Eller (1995), and Scott (1999) for empowering feminist perspectives on religion and spirituality.

Haldeman (1996) emphasizes the importance of separating from hostile religious institutions that inflict psychological damage. Separating themselves from oppressive religious institutions that are resolute in their anti-gay doctrine can be empowering for some lesbians. In most communities, especially larger urban areas, lesbian and gay inclusive religious services are available.

For lesbians who wish to maintain their connections to lifelong mainstream religious institutions, yet also challenge the heterosexism perpetrated by those institutions, a number of religious-oriented advocacy groups are available. Examples of these groups include, Dignity (Catholic), Integrity (Episcopalian), More Light (Presbyterian), Affirmation (Mormon, also United Methodist), Friends for Lesbian and Gay Concerns (Quaker), Seventh Day Adventist Kinship International (Seventh Day Adventist), the World Congress of Gay and Lesbian Jewish Organizations for Jews (Jewish), and Evangelicals Concerned (evangelicals).

Other lesbians may seek to nurture their spirituality without attaching themselves to formal religious institutions. While the practice of religion typically involves adherence to an established set of beliefs (religious doctrine) and participation in an organized community of others who ascribe to similar beliefs, the practice of spirituality relates more to individual experience and meaning-making of the divine (Van Hook, Hugen, & Aguilar, 2001). For more information on lesbian spirituality, the reader is referred to Lake (2001) and Van Dyke (1992).

IMPLICATIONS FOR HELPING PROFESSIONALS

Mainstream religion has epic heterosexist roots, and the trauma of religious oppression on the psychological health and well-being of lesbians should not be ignored in the therapeutic relationship. Religious beliefs should also be considered as an important component of understanding cultural diversity among lesbian clients (Shafranske & Maloney, 1996). The following suggestions may be useful for responding to religious and spirituality concerns expressed by lesbian clients:

1. *Evaluate the extent of religious trauma.* To what extent has the client been impacted by lesbian-negative religious doctrine? What specific experiences have occurred? How has religious oppression influenced client self-esteem, and how has it contributed to guilt, shame and internalized homophobia? Because low self-esteem and internalized homophobia can become risk factors for depression, suicidality, and substance abuse, these issues must be addressed in the counseling relationship.
2. *Honor losses engendered by religious oppression.* What losses (e.g., marginalization by or rejection from one's community of faith, rejection by one's family based on religious beliefs) has the client encountered? What has been the impact of those losses? Naming loss for what it is, and the trauma it evokes, can be an initial step toward the process of healing.
3. *Address the impact of religion as a tool for social injustice toward lesbians.* To what extent have clients critically examined the intersection of

religion and sexual orientation in their own lives? Helping them evaluate religious doctrine and its potential for the social control of sexuality can be valuable. It is important that client self-determination with regard to religious beliefs be honored in this activity. The imposition of personal religious doctrine by therapists would be unethical. Rather, the goal is to help clients critically evaluate (and reconstruct if they so desire) their own religious beliefs in response to an ethical value of religious social justice for lesbians.

4. *Develop a list of religious and spiritual resources to share with clients.* For those clients who seek resources for religious and spiritual support, they may benefit from the following types of information: a list of local places of worship that are lesbian-affirming; a list of lesbian-affirming religious and spiritual groups such as those that were noted earlier in this article; a referral list of area lesbian-affirming clergy who are willing to discuss religion and spirituality; and, a reading list of lesbian-affirming theology and spirituality (e.g., Christ, 1998; Christ & Plaskow, 1992; Eller, 1995; Lake, 2001; Johnson, 1992; Roscoe, 1988; Scott, 1999; Spong, 1988, 1991, 1998; Thistlewhite, 1991; Van Dyke, 1992).

CONCLUSION

While the social institution of religion has, indeed, engendered trauma in the lives of so many lesbians, the reality is that the once impregnable walls of religious intolerance are being stressed as never before. Oppressive religious doctrine, once unquestioned, is being challenged in the name of social justice for all people, regardless of sexual orientation. The means through which religious dogmatism has sought to control social order based on cultural prejudice–rather than on love and acceptance for all–are increasingly less tolerated by more and more faithful people of all creeds, races, and sexual orientations. And, the move toward social justice with regard to religion and sexual orientation is now a dynamic force whose voice will no longer be silenced.

REFERENCES

Akabas, S. H. (1995). The world of work. In N. Van Den Berg (Ed.), *Feminist practice in the 21st century* (pp. 105-125). Washington, D.C.: NASW Press.

Appleby, G. A., & Anastas, J. W. (1998). *Not just a passing phase: Social work with gay, lesbian, and bisexual people.* New York: Columbia.

Bailey, J. M., & Pillard, R. C. (1991). A genetic study of male sexual orientation. *Archives of General Psychiatry, 48*, 1089-1095.

Bailey, J. M., Pillard, R. C., Neale, M. C., & Agyei, Y. (1993). Heritable factors influence sexual orientation in women. *Archives of General Psychiatry, 50*, 217-223.

Bennett, L. (1998). *Mixed blessings: Organized religion and gay and lesbian Americans in 1998*. Washington, D.C.: Human Rights Campaign Fund.

Bordisso, L. A. (1988). *The relationship between level of moral development and sexual orientation by Roman Catholic priests*. Unpublished doctoral dissertation, University of San Francisco.

Boykin, K. (1996). *One more river to cross: Black and gay in America*. New York: Doubleday.

Cass, V. C. (1979). Homosexual identity formation: A theoretical model. *Journal of Homosexuality, 4*(3), 219-235.

Cass, V. C. (1984a). Homosexual identity: A concept in need of definition. *Journal of Homosexuality, 9*(2/3), 105-126.

Cass, V. C. (1984b). Homosexual identity formation: Testing a theoretical model. *Journal of Sex Research, 20*(2), 143-167.

Christ, C. P. (Ed.). (1998). *Rebirth of the Goddess: Finding meaning in feminist spirituality*. New York: Routledge.

Christ, C. P., & Plaskow, J. (Eds.). (1992). *Womanspirit rising: A feminist reader in religion*. San Francisco: Harper.

Clark, J. M., Brown, J. C., & Hochstein, L. M. (1989). Institutional religion and gay/lesbian oppression. *Marriage and Family Review, 14*(3-4), 265-284.

Creech, J. (1998). *Response to the judicial charge*. Omaha, NE, First United Methodist Church.

Davidson, M. G. (2000). Religion and spirituality. In R. M. Perez & K. A. DeBord (Eds.), *Handbook of counseling and psychotherapy with lesbian, gay, and bisexual clients* (pp. 409-433).

Eller, C. (1995). *Living in the lap of the Goddess: The feminist spirituality movement in America*. Boston: Beacon Press.

Faludi, S. (1991). *Backlash: The undeclared war against American women*. New York: Crown.

Gomes, P. J. (1996). *The good book: Reading the Bible with heart and mind*. New York: William Morrow.

Haldeman, D. C. (1994). The practice and ethics of sexual orientation conversion therapy. *Journal of Consulting and Clinical Psychology, 62*(2), 221-227.

Haldeman, D. C. (1996). Spirituality and religion in the lives of lesbians and gay men. In R. P. Cabaj & T. S. Stein (Eds.), *Textbook of homosexuality and mental health* (pp. 881-896). Washington, D.C.: American Psychiatric Association.

Hamer, D. H., Hu, S., Magnuson, V. L., Hu, N., & Pattatucci, A. M. (1993). A linkage between DNA markers on the X chromosome and male sexual orientation. *Science, 261*, 321-327.

Heyward, C. (1989). *Speaking of Christ: A lesbian feminist voice*. New York: Pilgrim Press.

Hilton, B. (1992). *Can homophobia be cured?* Nashville, TN: Abingdon.

Holy Bible (New Revised Standard Version). (1989). Grand Rapids, MI: Zondervan Publishing House.

Human Rights Campaign. (1999). *Mission impossible: Why reparative therapy and ex-gay ministries fail*. Human Rights Campaign Foundation.

Johnson, W. R. (1992). Protestantism and gay and lesbian freedom. In B. Berson (Ed.), *Positively gay: New approaches to gay and lesbian life* (2nd ed.) (pp. 210-232). Berkeley, CA: Celestial Arts.

Lake, C. (Ed.). (2001). *Recreations: Religion and spirituality in the lives of queer people*. Ontario, CA: Insomniac Group.

LeVay, S. (1991). A difference in hypothalamic structure between heterosexual and homosexual men. *Science, 253*, 1034-1037.

Mahaffy, K. A. (1996). Cognitive dissonance and its resolution: A study of lesbian Christians. *Journal for the Scientific Study of Religion, 35*(4), 392-402.

McNeill, J. J. (1993). *The church and the homosexual* (4th ed.). New York: Beacon.

Mitchell, H. R. (1983). Moral development and sexual orientation. *Dissertation Abstracts International, 44*, 4412A.

More Light Presbyterians of Charlotte. (2001). *Reflections, 2*(2), 2. Author.

Morrow, D. F. (1996). Heterosexism: Hidden discrimination in social work education. *Journal of Gay and Lesbian Social Services, 5*(4), 1-16.

Popple, P. R., & Leighninger, L. (2002). *Social work, social welfare, and American society* (5th ed.). Boston: Allyn & Bacon.

Ritter, K. Y., & O'Neill, C. W. (1989). Moving through loss: The spiritual journey of gay men and lesbian women. *Journal of Counseling and Development, 68*, 9-15.

Rodriguez, E. M., & Ouellette, S. C. (2000). Gay and lesbian Christians: Homosexual and religious identity integration in the members and participants of a gay-positive church. *Journal for the Scientific Study of Religion, 39*(3), 333-348.

Roscoe, W. (Ed.). (1988). *Living the spirit: A gay American Indian anthology*. New York: St. Martin's.

Scott, I. C. (1999). *God is a woman: The last taboo and hidden secrets at the millennium*. Greyden Press.

Shafranske, E. P., & Maloney, H. N. (1996). Religion and the clinical practice of psychology: A case for inclusion. In E. P. Shafranske (Ed.), *Religion and the clinical practice of psychology*. Washington, D.C.: American Psychological Association.

Shuck, K. D., & Liddle, B. J. (2001). Religious conflicts experienced by lesbian, gay, and bisexual individuals. *Journal of Gay and Lesbian Psychotherapy, 5*(2), 2001.

Singer, B. L., & Deschamps, D. (1994). *Gay and lesbian stats: A pocket guide of facts and figures*. New York: Harper Collins.

Spong, J. S. (1988). *Living in sin? A bishop rethinks sexuality*. Nashville, TN: Abingdon.

Spong, J. S. (1991). *Rescuing the Bible from fundamentalism*. San Francisco: Harper & Row.

Spong, J. S. (1998). *Why Christianity must change or die*. San Francisco: Harper.

Taylor, T. S. (2000). Is God good for you, good for your neighbor? The influence of religious orientation on demoralization and attitudes toward lesbians and gay men. *Dissertation Abstracts International, 60*(12-A), 4472.

Thistlewhite, S. (1991). *Sex, race, and God: Christian feminism in black and white*. New York: Crossroad.

Thompson, E. H. (1991). Beneath the status characteristic: Gender variations in religiousness. *Journal for the Scientific Study of Religion, 30*(4), 333-347.

Van Dyke, A. (1992). *The search for a woman-centered spirituality: The cutting edge: Lesbian life and literature*. New York: New York University Press.

Van Hook, M., Hugen, B., & Aguilar, M. (Eds.). (2001). *Spirituality within religious traditions in social work practice*. Pacific Grove, CA: Brooks/Cole.

White, M. (1995). *Stranger at the gate: To be gay and Christian in America*. Plume.

Community Interventions Concerning Homophobic Violence and Partner Violence Against Lesbians

Suzanna M. Rose

SUMMARY. Homophobic violence and same-sex domestic violence against lesbians are described in this paper based on survey research and hotline calls conducted by a community anti-violence project. A community survey of 229 lesbians indicated that during a one-year period, about fifteen percent had been the target of homophobic violence and twelve percent had been the victim of same-sex partner violence. Violence was defined as including assault with a weapon, physical assault, sexual assault, stalking, and property destruction. The prevalence study was contrasted with actual hotline calls from lesbians during a five-year

Suzanna M. Rose, PhD, is Professor of Psychology and Director of the Women's Studies Center at Florida International University. Dr. Rose's research focuses on relationships and sexuality as well on the victimization of lesbians and gay men. She is on the Editorial Boards of *Psychology of Women Quarterly, Sex Roles, Women & Therapy*, and the American Psychological Association/Division 44 series on *Contemporary Perspectives on Lesbian, Gay, and Bisexual Psychology*. She also is a member of the grant review panel for the American Psychological Foundation Wayne Placek Award for research on lesbian and gay issues.

Address correspondence to: Suzanna M. Rose, PhD, Women's Studies Center, DM212, Florida International University, Miami, FL 33199 (E-mail: srose@fiu.edu).

[Haworth co-indexing entry note]: "Community Interventions Concerning Homophobic Violence and Partner Violence Against Lesbians." Rose, Suzanna M. Co-published simultaneously in *Journal of Lesbian Studies* (Harrington Park Press, an imprint of The Haworth Press, Inc.) Vol. 7, No. 4, 2003, pp. 125-139; and: *Trauma, Stress, and Resilience Among Sexual Minority Women: Rising Like the Phoenix* (ed: Kimberly F. Balsam) Harrington Park Press, an imprint of The Haworth Press, Inc., 2003, pp. 125-139. Single or multiple copies of this article are available for a fee from The Haworth Document Delivery Service [1-800-HAWORTH, 9:00 a.m. - 5:00 p.m. (EST). E-mail address: docdelivery@haworthpress.com].

http://www.haworthpress.com/store/product.asp?sku=J155

10.1300/J155v07n04_08

period. Examples illustrate how interventions based on these findings were used to influence police response, victim services, and legislation.

KEYWORDS. Lesbian, homophobic violence, hate crimes, bias crimes, same-sex domestic violence, intimate partner violence, domestic violence, community intervention

Homophobic hate crime victimization and same-sex partner violence are two types of violence known to affect lesbians that recently have begun to receive attention from researchers, mental health providers, and policy makers. Homophobic violence refers to harassment or assault that is based on prejudice concerning the victim's actual or perceived sexual orientation (Berrill, 1992). Homophobic violence is widespread, with estimates indicating that one in five lesbians have been assaulted in an anti-lesbian incident in their lifetime (e.g., Herek, Gillis, & Cogan, 1999). Less is known about the prevalence of lesbian partner violence, but some research suggests that domestic violence is about as common in lesbian relationships as in heterosexual ones, with one in five lesbians experiencing at least one incident (e.g., West, 2002).

In response to anti-lesbian (as well as anti-gay) victimization, many communities have established anti-violence projects. Across the U.S. during the past decade, 24 to 30 anti-violence projects have operated annually to document hate crimes under the umbrella of the National Coalition of Anti-Violence Programs (NCAVP, 2001a). A smaller number of these programs also provide domestic violence services (NCAVP, 2001b). These organizations aim to increase general public awareness of violence against and within the lesbian, gay, bisexual and transgendered community, provide services to victims, and advocate for social, legal, and policy reforms that would better protect sexual minorities.

The goals in the present paper are twofold. The first is to describe homophobic violence and same-sex domestic violence against lesbians based on the findings of an urban lesbian and gay anti-violence project. The results of community survey research and hotline calls will be used to describe prevalence and case studies of each type of violence. The second goal is to illustrate how interventions based on these sources were used to influence police response, victim services, and legislation.

THE LESBIAN AND GAY ANTI-VIOLENCE PROJECT

The community organization described here, the St. Louis Lesbian and Gay Anti-Violence Project (AVP),[1] operated from 1992 to 2000. During that time, the St. Louis AVP was a member of the National Coalition of Anti-Violence Programs and participated in a national tracking project concerning hate crimes and same-sex domestic violence. As cofounder and director of the AVP, the author helped to develop the crisis counseling services and data collection procedures. Over time, the opportunities increased for the AVP to interact with victim service agencies, police and the courts, community boards, and legislators. It quickly became apparent that documenting and responding to hate and same-sex domestic violence could serve a vital function in bringing about social change. Similar to some programs in other cities, the AVP rose to this challenge by conducting community surveys to assess the prevalence of violence as well as by providing direct services to victims through a hotline.

Prevalence of Violence Against Lesbians

A major issue that the AVP confronted continually was the lack of awareness concerning lesbians as victims of violence among both the lesbian and gay community and the larger heterosexual and law enforcement community. The prevailing stereotype was that gay men were the natural and most frequent targets of homophobic hate crime. In addition, a strong belief predominated that lesbians seldom engaged in domestic violence. These stereotypes are common in the U.S. and typically pose problems for effective community intervention (cf., McLaughlin & Rozee, 2001; Ristock, 2001). The stereotype was supported to some extent by prevalence studies indicating that gay men more often than lesbians are the victims of most types of physical violence and intimidation based on sexual orientation (cf., Berrill, 1992; Herek et al., 1999). In addition, because men more often than women are the perpetrators of physical assaults (Tjaden & Thoennes, 2000), it is understandable that people might expect men more often than women to be violent in same-sex relationships.

Contrary to this perception, research shows that many lesbians are indeed the target of both homophobic violence and domestic violence. From 12% to 19% of lesbians have experienced anti-lesbian hate crime victimization as an adult at least once (von Schultess, 1992; Herek et al., 1999). Among 980 lesbian participants studied recently by Herek and colleagues (1999), property crimes were reported most often (9%), followed by physical assault (7%), attempted physical assault (6%), sexual assault (3%), attempted sexual assault (2%), and robbery (1%). In terms of intimate partner violence, estimates have ranged from 11% to 45% (e.g., Tjaden & Thoennes, 2000; Waldner-Haugrud,

Gratch, & Magruder, 1997). The lower estimate of 11% was based on the percent of women experiencing rape, physical assault or stalking from a cohabiting woman partner reported in a national survey of violence against women (Tjaden & Thoennes, 2000). The higher estimate of 45% was found by Waldner-Haugrud and colleagues (1997) who examined victimization by a lesbian partner using a broader range of behaviors, including threats, pushing, slapping, punching, being struck with an object, or use of a weapon.

Survey Method and Results

Like other intervention programs, our group faced the need to verify that similar problems existed specifically within our community. Thus, the AVP conducted several community surveys focusing on the prevalence of homophobic and same-sex partner violence and related issues among lesbians and gay men in the St. Louis metropolitan area. A secondary educational goal also was satisfied by providing participants with information about AVP services at the end of the survey. The survey described in the present study was distributed at one gay pride event. A shady rest area was provided for participants to complete the survey.

The AVP developed the Community Needs Assessment Survey to assess the prevalence of homophobic and same-sex violence against lesbians and gay men. Survey questions focused on participants' knowledge about the AVP, as well as extent of harassment and violence in the past year resulting from homophobic and same-sex partner incidents. The findings reported in the present study pertain only to the subset of questions that assessed physical violence aimed at lesbians. Participants were asked if they had experienced assault with a weapon, sexual assault, physical assault, stalking, or property destruction during the past year in the context of either (a) an anti-lesbian/gay incident, or (b) violence from a same-sex partner. Additional questions assessed demographic characteristics, including gender (female, male, transgendered); age, sexual orientation (gay/lesbian, bisexual or heterosexual); and race and education (open-ended). Also assessed was (a) the degree to which the participant was "out" (i.e., "Please indicate the extent to which you are 'out' as a lesbian/gay/bisexual/transgendered person") using an 8-point Likert scale, not at all out (0) to completely out (7), and (b) the degree of involvement in community organizations (i.e., "How would you describe your level of involvement in lesbian/gay/bisexual/transgendered community organizations?") using a 4-point scale, not at all active/involved (0), very active/involved (3).

The Community Needs Assessment Survey was completed by 563 participants. Of these, 32 heterosexual, 56 bisexual, and 4 respondents who did not specify their sexual orientation were dropped from the sample. The resulting final sample was comprised of 229 lesbians and 242 gay men. The results pertaining to five questions concerning physical violence from the 229 lesbian participants are reported below. The lesbian participants were between 16 and 65 years of age, with a mean age of 30 (*SD* = 8.01 years). The majority were White (79%) and most had a minimum of some college education (85%). The participants reported being "somewhat out" to "mostly out" in terms of their sexual orientation (*M* = 5.4, *SD* = .10; 7 = completely out) and indicated that on average, they were "somewhat active or involved" (*M* = 1.2, *SD* = .06; 3 = very active/involved) in lesbian and gay community organizations.

As shown in Table 1, 15% of participants reported having been the target of at least one act of anti-lesbian bias violence and 12% indicated experiencing at least one act of physical violence in a same-sex relationships during the past year. Because of the way responses were elicited (i.e., using a checklist), it is possible that more than one violent behavior may have occurred during a single incident. Types of violence occurring during bias incidents most often included homophobic stalking (16%) and property destruction (13%). Other violent bias acts included sexual assault (7%), physical assault (5%), and assault with a weapon (2%). In terms of same-sex partner violence, the most often reported behaviors included property destruction (10%), physical assault (9%), and stalking (7%). Sexual assault and assault with a weapon by a partner were reported infrequently (< 3%).

The results of the AVP Community Needs Assessment Survey provided a basis for opening a discussion with community leaders, local media, and police concerning violence against lesbians and gay men. The finding that from twelve to fifteen percent of lesbians experienced serious homophobic or domestic violence in a one-year period was newsworthy. However, we acknowledged that the prevalence of violence obtained from a convenience sample

TABLE 1. Percentage of Lesbians Reporting Crime Victimization from Homophobic and Partner Violence During the Past Year

	Crime Victimization in Past Year (%) (*N* = 229)	
Type of Victimization	Homophobic Violence	Partner Violence
One or more incident	**15.4**	**12.2**
Stalking	16.6	7.4
Property destruction	13.1	10.0
Sexual assault	7.4	2.2
Physical assault	5.2	8.7
Assault with a weapon	1.7	2.6

may have been overestimated, since individuals who attend a gay pride event may be more open about their sexual orientation and thus more vulnerable to bias incidents.

We made projections based on the survey that were calculated in the following way. The size of the metropolitan population served by the AVP was about 1,000,000. It was expected that as many as 30,000 women within that population might be lesbians based on a conservative estimate of 3% (Laumann, Gagnon, Michael, & Michaels, 1994). If 12% to 15% of those experienced homophobic or same-sex partner violence annually as suggested by the community survey, the volume of incidents involving lesbians might range from 3,600 to 4,500. We indicated that these projections might be an overestimate and should be interpreted with caution. Nevertheless, the projected figures provided a compelling argument for increased community and law enforcement support for unacknowledged or hidden victims. The local print media picked up on the survey results and produced several articles focusing on lesbian and gay hate crimes and domestic violence.

Case Studies of Violence Against Lesbians: Hotline Calls

The AVP hotline operated from 2 p.m. to 10 p.m. daily using a paging system. The AVP volunteer on call was paged when a hotline report came in and returned the call immediately. The volunteer then took an extensive report of the incident and provided crisis counseling, referrals, and if possible, intervention. Reports based on hotline calls functioned in two important ways for the AVP. First, in combination with the community survey, they showed that lesbian victims of violence were being underserved. For instance, during the five-year period from 1995-1999, lesbians made a total of 104 calls to the AVP Hotline concerning homophobic violence and same-sex partner violence. Seventy-eight calls were reports of anti-lesbian violence and 26 concerned lesbian partner violence. The low number of hotline calls relative to the estimates of violence projected from survey results indicated that the victimization of lesbians was not being adequately addressed.

A second way that hotline calls had an important impact was in terms of the specific case study examples they provided. Case examples were the most potent way to address the general invisibility of lesbians as victims. They also were particularly useful for working with victim services, the police, and legislators because they demonstrated where services or effective intervention were lacking or showed the need for greater response and legal protection.

Case examples of five types of incidents (assault with a weapon, physical assault, sexual assault, stalking, and vandalism) taken from the 78 hotline calls concerning homophobic violence against lesbians are presented in Table 2. Likewise, case examples of five types of crimes taken from the 26 domestic violence calls are presented in Table 2.

In most of the case examples reported in Table 2, responses to the victims by police, the legal system, the media, and victim services were hostile, inadequate, or dismissive. For instance, in Case 1 concerning the murder of a lesbian by her partner's ex-husband, the case was sensationalized as a "love triangle." Newspaper accounts of the murder also made reference to a movie, *Heavenly Creatures*, about two lesbians who killed one of the girls' mothers because she tried to keep them apart, notwithstanding the fact that the two lesbians in the incident reported to the AVP were the victims, not the murderers. Police did not report the homicide as a hate crime and it was not prosecuted as a hate crime. At the trial, the defense attorney argued that the murder victim was "not a good person or mother" because she was a lesbian–an argument that was heard by one daughter of the murdered woman, who was present at the trial.

Inadequate or hostile police response was an issue in many cases. Victims reported being fearful of calling the police either because they feared police homophobia or because they feared retaliation from the perpetrator for reporting the incident. In Case 3, a hate crime incident, a lesbian who was sexually fondled by a male coworker was harassed by the police when she reported the incident. Although an arrest was made and the perpetrator was charged, the victim was fearful that the perpetrator might retaliate by physically assaulting her at some point. Her negative experience with the police added to her feelings of vulnerability, because she did not believe they would help her. In Case 7, a domestic violence incident, police who responded to the victim's 911 call concerning domestic violence made a decision to arrest both women. This is a common response among police when faced with same-sex domestic violence and one that causes considerable emotional and legal problems for the victim (NCAVP, 2001b). Moreover, the police taunted the victim about her sexuality when she was in jail and continued to harass her after her release.

In some instances, the police were not called and therefore did not intervene. For example, in Case 5, a lesbian was verbally harassed and her car was vandalized, but the victim, witnesses and security officers did not call the police. Similarly, in Case 6, involving a lesbian who had been seriously abused by her partner, the victim was afraid to call the police because she did not believe they would be able to stop her ex-partner from killing her. In Case 8, another domestic violence case, the victim expressed fear that reporting the violence or car theft to the police would escalate the violence. She also feared harassment from the police.

Victim services constituted another area where response to violence against lesbians was unavailable or inadequate. In two lesbian domestic violence

TABLE 2. Case Examples of Lesbian Hate Crime and Domestic Violence Hotline Calls

---

Hate Crimes

Case 1: Assault with a Weapon/Murder

A White, 34-year-old lesbian reported that her ex-husband had shot and killed her woman partner, a White woman, age 35.The ex-husband had confronted the two women in their home with a gun and shot the partner once in the face, then fired several more shots into her body.The ex-husband forced the client to take her partner's pulse so she would know her lover was dead. The ex-husband then reloaded the gun and handed it to the client and told her to kill herself.When the client refused, the ex-husband lunged at her and she shot and wounded him.

Case 2: Physical Assault

A 17-year-old, White lesbian and her girlfriend reported being attacked in a lesbian-bashing incident at their high school as they were walking into the school. Two young males jumped one of the women, threw her to the ground, and punched her six or seven times in the face. The assailants yelled homophobic insults, such as "Hey, you dykes." The client's girlfriend escaped, ran to the car, and pressed on the horn until the perpetrators ran away. The victim sustained a black eye and facial bruises and was robbed.

Case 3: Sexual Assault

An African American lesbian in her 30s reported being sexually assaulted at her workplace by a male coworker. He put his hands under her clothes, fondled her, and pressed up against her while making such comments as, "You're too pretty to be gay." The perpetrator was arrested and charged with a misdemeanor sexual offense. The client reported harassment from the police, with one police officer saying, "Why are you doing this to this man? He just patted you on the butt. What were you wearing? What did you do to encourage him?" Coworkers made similar comments. The perpetrator was fired, and the client quit her job after the incident. She reported feeling "dirty, disillusioned, and afraid." She was also concerned that the assailant might "jump me in a parking lot. He beats his girlfriend. Who knows how far he's willing to go?"

Case 4: Stalking

Two White lesbians in their 40s reported being harassed repeatedly for more than two years by a woman who sent anti-lesbian letters to the victims' home, workplaces, and neighbors. The messages named the victims, revealed their sexual orientation, claimed they were a danger to the community, and demanded that they be fired from their jobs. One of the victims was a schoolteacher whose job was jeopardized by these actions. Although the women moved to a new neighborhood and took new jobs recently, the perpetrator had begun a rash of letters and phone calls to both the new neighbors and jobs.

Case 5: Property Destruction

A White lesbian in her 40s was harassed by a man at a local medical clinic. The harasser called her a "Lezzie" in a loud and hostile manner. The victim ignored the man, but he continued to harass her, saying, "You must want to be treated like a man, because you want women and you dress like a man. Then I'll treat you like a man." He screamed "Lezzie" several times and yelled that he was going to "kick her ass." The clinic staff came out and Security was called, but took no action. In the following week, the client's car tires were slit and the man continued to harass her. Clinic staff told the victim to ignore the vandalism and harassment. A nurse who witnessed the initial incident told the victim that she'd asked for it [the violence] by being "out."

Domestic Violence

Case 6: Assault with a Weapon

An African American lesbian in her thirties was being threatened by her ex-partner, an African American woman also in her thirties, who had violently abused her during their relationship of one year (her first lesbian relationship). The partner was threatening to kill the client, who had moved out the day of the call. The perpetrator previously had beaten the client in the face and arms, had burned and cut her with a knife, and had broken her pelvis. She had been hospitalized for these injuries in the past. The perpetrator was a drug dealer and the client believed that no one would be able to stop the partner from killing her. The client's partner also had called her at work and threatened her.

Case 7: Physical Assault

The client, a White lesbian (age unknown), reported domestic violence and harassment from her white, female partner (age unknown). During the most recent incident, the partner pinned the client down and punched her very hard in the back of the neck. The client called the police, but when they arrived, they arrested both her and her partner. The police did not check for any prior police record or they would have learned that the partner had a prior felony conviction. The perpetrator later claimed that she was the victim and obtained a restraining order against the client. When the perpetrator came to the house to remove her belongings, the police officers accompanying her harassed the client, asking, "How did you like the inside of our jail?"

Case 8: Sexual Assault

A White lesbian (age unknown) reported that her current woman partner (age, race unknown) of two years was emotionally and physically abusive. She reported more than 10 previous incidents resulting in minor injury.The abuser would slap the client and pinch her breasts when coercing her to have sex. The abuser had also taken possession of the client's car. The client wanted to end the relationship but wasn't sure how to do it, because her partner had keys to her apartment. She was afraid to change the locks or report the car theft to the police.

Case 9: Stalking

A White lesbian (age 45-64) reported that her former White woman partner (age 45-64) had been stalking her since the client left their 10-year relationship. The client reported repeated abuse by her ex-partner, including being set on fire by her. The client had a restraining order against her ex-partner, but was feeling drawn towards her since a recent phone conversation.

Case 10: Property Destruction

A White lesbian (age 35) called to report that her partner, a White lesbian (age 30-44), was being emotionally, verbally, and physically abusive to her and verbally abusive to her 4-year-old son. The relationship always was difficult but had gotten worse since the client was accepted into nursing school and was due to begin in 3 weeks. Recently, the client went out and didn't come home all night. When she returned, she found that her partner had broken her 4-year-old son's rifle gun and racetrack and had verbally abused the boy. The partner was drinking more and was becoming more unpredictable. Both the client and partner used cocaine occasionally.

---

cases, Case 9 and Case 10, victims were unable to find established shelters or agencies where the staff were able to provide lesbians with safety and sensitive help. The lesbian in Case 9 who had been abused and stalked by her ex-partner and was feeling drawn into the relationship again had called two local women's shelters and asked if they had a lesbian counselor on staff, but was told they did not. This client wanted to talk to someone who understood lesbian relationships. In Case 10, the lesbian whose partner had broken her son's toys was seeking shelter but wanted to know if any shelters "specialized" in lesbians, because she didn't want to have to deal with the homophobia of other shelter clients. None of the shelters in the region had any specialized services for lesbians, however.

A lack of protective legislation concerning hate crimes based on sexual orientation was a limiting factor in responding to other cases. For example, police could not intervene in Case 4, involving the homophobic mail and telephone stalking of a lesbian couple, because the perpetrator had not threatened any violence or physical harm to the victims. However, since the perpetrator lived in another state, the victims reported it as a hate crime to the civil right bureau of the FBI, which has jurisdiction over hate crimes that cross state lines. Unfortunately, the FBI agent was not able to investigate because hate crimes based on sexual orientation were not covered by federal hate crime legislation; thus, the incident was outside his sphere of authority.

In sum, the survey indicated that both homophobic hate crimes and domestic violence incidents were prevalent among lesbians in the metropolitan area served by the AVP. Types of incidents included assault with a weapon, physical assault, sexual assault, stalking, and property destruction. In addition, hotline calls added depth to the nature of such incidents and revealed specific areas in which community intervention might improve police response, victim services, and legislation.

COMMUNITY INTERVENTIONS

In response to the limitations in responding to violence against lesbians described above, the AVP successfully implemented three community interventions. The first intervention was aimed at increasing police responsiveness to violence against lesbians and involved working closely with key officials within the police department. A major improvement in relations between the police and the lesbian and gay community occurred after several meetings between police captains and the AVP, when one captain[2] agreed to serve as a liaison to the lesbian and gay community. Having a liaison made it possible for the AVP to mediate between victims and the police. For instance, in incidents similar to Case 5, in which police harassment of a lesbian victim of vandalism occurred, the AVP would contact the police liaison, who in turn would investigate the responding officer's treatment of the victim and, if necessary, bring the unprofessional conduct to the attention of the officer's superior.

Another important improvement occurred when the police liaison proposed a system of "soft reporting" of crimes against lesbians and gay men via AVP intervention. In soft reporting, the AVP would respond to calls concerning assaults by informing the police liaison, who would then call the victim, take a report, and take appropriate police action. Thus, lesbian victims did not have to call 911 and possibly face unsympathetic or homophobic police officers. This allowed for immediate response to some domestic violence calls that were made to the hotline while the abuse was in progress. In those cases, the police liaison dispatched hand-selected officers to the site who were able to apprehend the perpetrator.

Another type of soft reporting that was helpful to domestic violence victims involved the Domestic Violence Assault Team (DART). The police liaison had paved the way for the AVP to conduct a training session with DART concerning how to respond to lesbian and gay domestic violence incidents. Issues that were covered included: (a) how to identify whether an incident was intimate partner violence versus "roommate" violence (e.g., look at photographs to see if a same-sex couple relationship was evident; notice if the home had only one bedroom) and (b) how to avoid stereotyping when determining who was the aggressor (e.g., do not assume that the larger or stronger individual is the aggressor; do not resort to mutual arrest just because the incident involves individuals of the same-sex). This training led to stronger connections with DART officers who were very supportive of soft reporting by the AVP. For example, in Case 6, involving domestic violence with a weapon and physical assault, the AVP called DART and reported the incident. The responding DART officer then called the victim, took a report, and helped the victim obtain a restraining order. The DART officer also called the perpetrator and warned her that the police would respond to further threats or assaults immediately.

The second community intervention undertaken by the AVP involved working with victim service agencies to make them more aware of lesbian and gay issues. This intervention was facilitated when the AVP director (and author) was appointed to the St. Louis County Family and Domestic Violence Council[3] by St. Louis County Commissioners. The FDVC was an umbrella organization comprised of judges, lawyers, and victim service representatives whose mission was to improve law enforcement response to domestic violence in St. Louis County. Through the FDVC, the AVP became involved in training victim service volunteers and staff that led to two improvements. The first concerned intakes and treatment at victim service agencies. Volunteers and staff were sensitized concerning how to be alert to possible lesbian domestic violence victims (e.g., be alert when callers refer to a gender-unspecified "partner"; do not automatically insert "he" or assume that the perpetrator is male when speaking to callers). In addition, the AVP was able to work with selected agencies to identify staff who could serve as specialists in lesbian domestic violence. Agencies that did not have this capability were encouraged to refer lesbian clients to the AVP for supportive counseling.

Another improvement related to victim service agencies focused on increasing the accuracy of reporting concerning lesbian domestic violence. The victim service organizations affiliated with the FDVC were receiving calls from lesbian clients but not documenting them separately. The AVP, as a member of the NCAVP national tracking program for lesbian and gay domestic violence, was invested in reporting such incidents but received relatively few calls from domestic violence victims. Thus, an arrangement was made between the AVP and two agencies for each agency to record and forward the information concerning lesbian domestic violence cases to the AVP on a monthly basis.

The third community intervention by the AVP was aimed at legislators. As reported in Case 4, the absence of protective hate crime legislation encompassing sexual orientation was a barrier to effective police and criminal justice intervention at the federal level. A lack of protection at the state level was equally a problem. In response, the AVP worked closely with two organizations to have sexual orientation included in the Missouri hate crimes law. The first organization was the Privacy Rights Education Project (PREP), a lobby group whose mission was to pass legislation that would prevent discrimination based on sexual orientation and to repeal laws already on the books that were discriminatory. PREP[4] had been working with key legislators in Missouri[5] to propose a new hate crime bill. The second organization was the U.S. Attorney Generals' Hate Crimes Task Force for Missouri-Illinois. The Hate Crimes Task Force was comprised of the two U.S. Attorney Generals for Eastern Missouri and Southern Illinois, as well as representatives from police departments, the FBI, and appointed members of various advocacy groups, including the AVP, Urban League, Anti-Defamation League, National Alliance of Christians and Jews, Paraquad (an advocacy group for persons with disabilities), and others.

A presentation by the AVP using cases of hate crime victimization against lesbians and gay men in St. Louis helped to persuade the Hate Crimes Task Force to endorse a proposed change in the former Missouri Ethnic Intimidation Act. The proposed change would add sexual orientation, sex, and disability to the protected categories. The Hate Crimes Task Force was perceived to be an important ally because it was comprised of law enforcement groups that supported the new bill. In addition, the AVP identified lesbian and gay hate crime victims who went to the state capitol to provide victim testimony to the legislature. The AVP also provided survey results concerning hate crime prevalence that was used by PREP in its lobbying efforts.

Our joint effort to pass a new Hate Crime Bill was successful on May 14, 1999. The new law passed by the Missouri legislature represented a major victory for lesbian, gay, bisexual, and transgendered civil rights. The bill added sexual orientation, sex, and disability to the categories covered by the former Ethnic Intimidation Act and allowed extra penalties to be applied to hate crimes. Governor Carnahan later signed the bill into law. Of the 22 states that introduced similar bills in 1999, Missouri's hate crime bill was the only one to have passed. At the time, only 20 other states included sexual orientation in their hate crime laws.

In sum, community interventions undertaken by the AVP were successful due to several factors. First, the prevalence findings concerning homophobic and partner violence against lesbians provided evidence that was useful in convincing the police, victim services agencies, and legislators that a serious problem existed. Next, case studies enabled the AVP to personalize these events and elicit sympathy and sometimes outrage about injustices that were helpful in mobilizing people to action. Last, the survey and hotline results legitimized the activities of the AVP and enabled its representatives to become spokespersons of the lesbian and gay community within important institutions.

CONCLUSION

Homophobic and partner violence against lesbians continue to be relatively "low profile" events in both the lesbian and gay community and society at large. However, the lack of awareness can be addressed effectively by collecting evidence concerning both the extent of the problem and the details of individual cases. The efforts of the AVP described here illustrate that a combination of traditional survey research and case examples are strong educational tools for raising awareness about violence against lesbians. Community interventions based on these sources of information can be used successfully to influence police, victim services, and legislation.

Research on hate crimes and same-sex partner violence is in its early stages and has focused primarily on prevalence. However, future research should aim to determine the features and psychological consequences of these incidents. Recent research by Herek and colleagues (1999; 2002) and Rose and Mechanic (2002) have begun to provide more systematic descriptions of bias crimes. However, more evidence is needed concerning the crime features, psychological consequences, and help-seeking behaviors involved in both hate crimes and same-sex domestic violence.

NOTES

1. The author extends deepest appreciation to the following for their help in founding and supporting the St. Louis AVP: Barbara Brown, Mary Brown, Dayna Deck, James Dillon, Brian Edmiston, Matt Jorgenson, Leslie Kimball, Kris Kleindienst, Deke Law, Scott Emanuel, Mindy Mechanic, Ellen Tetlow, and Maria Whitter. Special thanks also is given to Blue Max, Challenge Metro, and MoKaBe's coffeehouse for their financial and moral support.

2. Gratitude is extended to Captain Joseph Richardson, St. Louis Police Department, for his advocacy concerning lesbian and gay victims of violence, his commitment to social justice, and his professionalism as a police officer. The author also thanks Clarence Harmon, former Mayor and Chief of Police.

3. The support of Judge Melvyn Weisman, Cathy Tofall, Director, Victim Services, and Barbara Bennett, Director, Women's Support and Community Services, was deeply appreciated.

4. Special thanks is extended to Jeff Wunrow, PREP's executive director, who spent long hours in Jefferson City negotiating the bill through the legislature; to Maria Whitter, PREP intern and former AVP member, who devoted every Tuesday to lobbying for the bill; and to the victims/survivors who provided their stories.

5. Lead sponsors were Senator William Clay, Jr. (D-St. Louis) and Rep. Tim Harlan (D Columbia). Also instrumental in helping pass the bill were Joan Bray (D-University City), openly gay Representative Tim Van Zant (D-Kansas City), Chuck Graham (D-Columbia), and John Dolan (R-Lake St. Louis).

REFERENCES

Berrill, K. T. (1992). Anti-gay violence and victimization in the United States: An overview. In G. M. Herek & K. T. Berrill (Eds.), *Hate crimes: Confronting violence against lesbians and gay men* (pp. 19-45). Newbury Park, CA: Sage.

Herek, G. M., Cogan, J. C., & Gillis, R. J. (2002). Victim experiences in hate crimes based on sexual orientation. *Journal of Social Issues*, *58*, 319-339.

Herek, G., Gillis, J. R., & Cogan, J. C. (1999). Psychological sequelae of hate crime victimization among lesbian, gay, and bisexual adults. *Journal of Consulting and Clinical Psychology*, *67*, 945-951.

Laumann, E. O., Gagnon, J. H., Michael, R. T., & Michaels, S. (1994). *The social organization of sexuality: Sexual practices in the United States*. Chicago: University of Chicago Press.

McLaughlin, E. M., & Rozee, P. D. (2001). Knowledge about heterosexual versus lesbian battering among lesbians. *Women and Therapy*, *23*, 39-58.

National Coalition of Anti-Violence Programs. (2001a). *Anti-lesbian/gay violence in the United States in 2000*. New York: Author.

National Coalition of Anti-Violence Programs. (2001b). *Lesbian, gay, transgender and bisexual domestic violence in 2000*. New York: Author.

Ristock, J. L. (2001). Decentering heterosexuality: Responses of feminist counselors to abuse in lesbian relationships. *Women and Therapy*, *23*, 59-72.

Rose, S. M., & Mechanic, M. (2002). Psychological distress, crime features, and help-seeking behaviors related to homophobic bias incidents. *American Behavioral Scientist, 46*(1), 14-26.

Tjaden, P., & Thoennes, N. (2000). Extent, nature, and consequences of intimate partner violence: Findings from the national violence against women survey. (NJ Report No. 118167). Washington, DC: U.S. Department of Justice.

Von Schultess, B. (1992). Violence in the streets: Anti-lesbian assault and harassment in San Francisco. In G. M. Herek & K. T. Berrill (Eds.), *Hate crimes: Confronting violence against lesbians and gay men* (pp. 65-75). Newbury Park: Sage.

Waldner-Haugrud, L. K., Vaden Gratch, L., & Magruder, B. (1997). Victimization and perpetration rates of violence in gay and lesbian relationships: Gender issues explored. *Violence and Victims, 12*, 173-184.

West, C. (2002). Lesbian intimate partner violence: Prevalence and dynamics. *Journal of Lesbian Studies, 6*, 119-125.

Index

Abuse
histories of, 56. *See also* Histories
physical. *See* Physical abuse
sexual. *See* Sexual abuse
Adjustment indicators, 21-25
African Methodist Episcopal Church, 115-118
Ages (self-identification), 10-11,16-17
American Psychiatric Association, 4-5
Anti-LBG (lesbian-bisexual-gay) victimization, 72, 74
AVP (Anti-Violence Project), 127-138

Balsam, K. F., 1-8,67-85
Behavior and emotional difficulties, 37-39
Biblical interpretations, 113-114
Black, A., 82-108
Black populations (multiple minority stress and resilience issues)
future perspectives of, 103-104
historical perspectives of, 88-89
insidious trauma, 90
introduction to, 87-89
MEES (mundane extreme environmental stress) experiences, 89-91,94
multicultural stress models, 89-90
multiple minority stress factors, 94-98
heterosexism, 95-97
identity fragmentation, 97-98
intersections (race-sexism-heterosexism), 97-98
racism, 94
sexism, 94-95
reference and research resources for, 103-108
resilience, 89,98-101
definition of, 89
emotional stability and management and, 99-100
external environmental contexts of, 98
internal self-characteristics of, 99-100
person-environment interaction processes of, 98-99
positive life outcomes of, 101
processes of, 100-101
self-esteem and, 99
socially supportive relationships and, 101
studies of, 88-104
analyses of, 92-93
discussion of, 102-103
goals and objectives of, 90-91
implications of, 102-103
introduction to, 88-89
limitations of, 103
measures for, 92
methods for, 91-93
participant data for, 91-92
procedures for, 91-92
results of, 92-101
theoretical frameworks for, 89-91
trustworthiness issues of, 93
Bowleg, L., 82-108
Brooks, K., 82-108
BSI (Brief Symptom Inventory), 14-15,72-73,76

Buffer effects (social support), 58
Burkholder, G., 82-108

Case studies (hotline calls), 130-134
Cass Model, 112-113
CDC (Centers for Disease Control), 50-51
CES-D (Center for Epidemiologic Studies Depression) Scale, 50,56
Christian religion issues, 109-123. *See also* Institutionalized Judeo-Christian religion issues
Church of God in Christ, 115-118
Church of Jesus Christ of Latter Day Saints, 115-118
"Coming out" process-related issues
  CSA (childhood sexual abuse) histories, 31-45
  disclosures in youth populations, 26
  emotional and behavior difficulties, 37-39
  future perspectives of, 45
  historical perspectives of, 31-33
  introduction to, 31-32
  reference and research resources for, 46-47
  sexuality feelings, 38-42
  studies of, 32-45
    discussion of, 42-45
    findings implications of, 44-45
    introduction to, 31-34
    limitations of, 43-44
    measures for, 35-36
    methods for, 34-36
    participant data for, 34-38
    procedures for, 36
    recruitment for, 34-35
    results of, 36-42
Community interventions (homophobic and partner violence-related issues)
  Ethnic Intimidation Act and, 137
  FBI (Federal Bureau of Investigation) and, 134
  future perspectives of, 137
  Hate Crime Bill and, 137-138
  Hate Crimes Task Force (U.S. Attorney General) and, 136
  historical perspectives of, 126-128
  introduction to, 125-126
  measures for, 128-137
    Community Needs Assessment Survey, 128-137
    introduction to, 128-130
  National Alliance of Christians and Jews and, 136
  NCAVP (National Coalition of Anti-Violence Programs) and, 126,131,136
  Paraquad and, 136
  reference and research resources for, 138-139
  St. Louis Lesbian and Gay AVP (Anti-Violence Project) and, 127-138
    community interventions of, 134-137
    DART (Domestic Violence Assault Team) of, 135-137
    hotline call case studies and, 130-134
    introduction to, 127
    participant data of, 129-130
    PREP (Property Rights Education Project) of, 136-138
    St. Louis County FDVC (Family and Domestic Violence Council) and, 135-137
    studies of, 128-134
    violence prevalence, 127-128
Community Needs Assessment Survey, 128-137
Community relationships, 14,20,26-27
Conservative Judaism, 115-118
Conversion therapy, 109,115,118
Cooperman, N. A., 49-66

Criticisms (research), 4
CSA (childhood sexual abuse)
  "coming out" process-related issues and, 31-45
  histories of, 31-45
  introduction to, 3
  victimization experiences and, 77-78

DART (Domestic Violence Assault Team), 135-137
D'Augelli, A. R., 9-29
Depression-related issues, 49-66. *See also* HIV-positive populations (abuse, support, and depression issues)
Developmental-related issues
  developmental challenges, 9-29. *See also* Youth populations (developmental challenges and victimization experiences)
  developmental contexts, 3-4
Disclosures, 26. *See also* "Coming-out" process-related issues
DSM-IV (Diagnostic and Statistical Manual, 4th edition), 4-5

Emotion-related issues
  emotional and behavior difficulties, 37-39
  emotional stability and management, 99-100
Empowerment and transformation issues, 118-119
Environmental-related issues
  environment-person interaction processes, 98-99
  external contexts, 98
Ethnic Intimidation Act, 137
Evangelical Lutheran Church of America, 115-118
External environmental contexts, 98

Family member victimization, 21
FBI (Federal Bureau of Investigation), 134
FDVC (Family and Domestic Violence Council), 135-137
Feelings (sexuality), 38-42
Fragmentation (identity), 97-98
Future perspectives
  of black populations (multiple minority stress and resilience issues), 103-104
  of "coming out" process-related issues, 45
  of community interventions (homophobic and partner violence-related issues), 137
  of HIV-positive populations (abuse, support, and depression issues), 63
  of institutionalized Judeo-Christian religion issues, 120
  of victimization experiences (mental health, revictimization, and sexual identity development issues), 82-83
  of youth populations (developmental challenges and victimization experiences), 27-28

GSI (Global Severity Index), 14-15, 22-24,72,76

Hate Crime Bill, 137-138
Hate Crimes Task Force (U.S. Attorney General), 136
Helping professional therapeutic relationships, 119-120
Heterosexism issues

Biblical interpretations, 113-114
heterosexism in religion, 111-113
heterosexism-sexism-race intersections, 97-98
multiple minority stress factors, 95-97
Historical perspectives
of black populations (multiple minority stress and resilience issues), 88-89
of "coming out" process-related issues, 31-33
of community interventions (homophobic and partner violence-related issues), 126-128
of HIV-positive populations (abuse, support, and depression issues), 50-55
of institutionalized Judeo-Christian religion issues, 110-111
of victimization experiences (mental health, revictimization, and sexual identity development issues), 68-70
Histories
of abuse, 56
of CSA (childhood sexual abuse), 31-45
HIV-positive populations (abuse, support, and depression issues)
CDC (Centers for Disease Control) and, 50-51
depression predictors, 57-58
future perspectives of, 63
historical perspectives of, 50-55
introduction to, 49-51
measures for, 50,53-57
abuse histories, 56
CES-D (Center for Epidemiologic Studies Depression) Scale, 50, 56
depressive symptomologies, 56
National Lesbian Health Care Survey, 53-55
sexual orientation, 57
social support, 56-57
UCLA Social Support Inventory, 56-57
physical abuse prevalence, 59-62
reference and research resources for, 63-66
risk factors, 51-52
depression, 52-55
among lesbian and bisexual women, 53-55
physical abuse, 51-55
sexual abuse, 51-55
social support and, 52-55
sexual abuse prevalence, 59-62
social support buffer effects, 58
studies of, 49-66
discussions of, 59-63
introduction to, 49-55
limitations of, 62-63
measures for, 56-57
methods of, 55-57
participant data for, 55,57
procedures for, 55
results, 57-59
sociodemographic data for, 58-59
Homophobic and partner violence-related issues, 125-139. *See also* Community interventions (homophobic and partner violence-related issues)
Hotline calls, 130-134
Huang, J., 82-108

Identity development issues
identity fragmentation, 97-98
identity integration, 112
victimization experiences, 67-85. *See also* Victimization experiences (mental health,

revictimization, and sexual identity development issues)
Injustices (social), 119-120
Insidious trauma, 90
Institutionalized Judeo-Christian religion issues
Biblical interpretations, 113-114
heterosexist interpretations, 113-114
introduction to, 113
literal interpretations, 113-114
conversion therapy, 109,115,118
future perspectives of, 120
helping professional therapeutic relationships, 119-120
introduction to, 119
religious and spiritual resources for, 120
religious oppression losses, 119
religious trauma evaluations, 119
social injustices and, 119-120
heterosexism in religion, 111-113
Cass Model and, 112-113
introduction to, 111-112
sexual orientation-religious identity integration, 112
historical perspectives of, 110-111
introduction to, 109-110
primary religious group positions, 114-118
African Methodist Episcopal Church, 115-118
Church of God in Christ, 115-118
Church of Jesus Christ of Latter Day Saints, 115-118
Evangelical Lutheran Church of America, 115-118
introduction to, 114-115
Judaism (Orthodox, Conservative, Reform, and Reconstructionist), 115-118
National Baptist Convention, 115-118
Roman Catholic Church, 115-118
Southern Baptist Convention, 115-118
United Methodist Church, 115-118
reference and research resources for, 120-123
religion as social institution, 110
sexism in religion, 110-111
transformation and empowerment, 118-119
Instruments (measurement). *See* Measures
Integration (sexual orientation-religious identity), 112
Interaction processes (person-environment), 98-99
Internal self-characteristics, 99-100
Interpretations (Biblical), 113-114
Intersections (race-sexist-hetero-sexism), 97-98

Judeo-Christian religion, 109-123. *See also* Institutionalized Judeo-Christian religion issues

Lesbian Wellness Survey, 71-72
Life outcomes (positive), 101
Lifetime victimization experiences, 14-15,20-21
Literal Biblical interpretations, 113-114
Litzenberger, B. W., 31-47
Lockhart, D. W., 49-66
Losses (religious oppression), 119

Measures
for black populations (multiple minority stress and resilience issues), 92

for "coming out" process-related issues, 35-36
for community interventions (homophobic and partner violence-related issues), 128-137
for HIV-positive populations (abuse, support, and depression issues), 50,53-57
instruments for, 14-15,22-24, 50-56,71-76,81,128-137
BSI (Brief Symptom Inventory), 14-15,72-73,76
CES-D (Center for Epidemiologic Studies Depression) Scale, 50,56
Community Needs Assessment Survey, 128-137
GSI (Global Severity Index), 14-15,22-24,72,76
Lesbian Wellness Survey, 71-72
National Lesbian Health Care Survey, 53-55,81
RSEI (Rosenberg Self-Esteem Inventory), 14-15
for victimization experiences (mental health, revictimization, and sexual identity development issues), 71-73
for youth populations (developmental challenges and victimization experiences), 12-16
MEES (mundane extreme environmental stress) experiences, 89-91,94
Models
Cass Model, 112-113
multicultural stress models, 89-90
Morris, J. F., 67-85
Morrow, D. F., 109-123
Multicultural stress models, 89-90
Multiple minority stress, 87-108. *See also* Black populations (multiple minority stress and resilience issues)

National Alliance of Christians and Jews, 136
National Baptist Convention, 115-118
National Lesbian Health Care Survey, 53-55,81
NCAVP (National Coalition of Anti-Violence Programs), 126,131,136

Oppression losses (religious), 119
Orthodox Judaism, 115-118

Paraquad, 136
Parental relationships, 13-14,17-20, 26-27
Partner and homophobic violence, 125-139. *See also* Community interventions (homophobic and partner violence-related issues)
Pearlman, L. A., 31-47
Person-environment interaction processes, 98-99
Physical abuse
prevalence of, 59-62
risk factors of, 51-55
victimization experiences, 74
Positive life outcomes, 101
Post-Traumatic Stress Disorder, 4-5
Predictors
of depression, 57-58
symptom, 10, 24
PREP (Property Rights Education Project), 136-138
Prevalence
of physical abuse, 59-62
of sexual abuse, 59-62
of violence, 127-128

Primary religious group positions, 114-118

Race- and ethnicity-related issues
multiple minority stress factors, 94
race-sexism-heterosexism intersections, 97-98
victimization experiences, 78
Reconstructionist Judaism, 115-118
Reference and research resources
for black populations (multiple minority stress and resilience issues), 103-108
for "coming out" process-related issues, 46-47
for community interventions (homophobic and partner violence-related issues), 138-139
for HIV-positive populations (abuse, support, and depression issues), 63-66
for institutionalized Judeo-Christian religion issues, 120-123
for victimization experiences (mental health, revictimization, and sexual identity development issues), 83-85
for youth populations (developmental challenges and victimization experiences), 28-29
Reform Judaism, 115-118
Relationships
parental, 13-14,17-20,26-27
socially supportive, 101
therapeutic, 119-120
Religious group positions, 114-118
Religious oppression losses, 119
Religious trauma evaluations, 119
Research
criticisms of, 4
resources. *See* Reference and research resources
studies. *See* Studies
Resilience
black populations (multiple minority stress and resilience issues), 89,98-101
definition of, 89
Revictimization, 76-77
Risk factors (HIV-positive populations), 51-52
Robohm, J. S., 31-47
Roman Catholic Church, 115-118
Rose, S. M., 125-139
RSEI (Rosenberg Self-Esteem Inventory), 14-15

Self-characteristics (internal), 99-100
Self-esteem, 99
Self-identification ages, 10-11,16-17
Sexism
multiple minority stress factors, 94-95
in religion, 110-111
sexism-heterosexism-race intersections, 97-98
Sexual abuse
prevalence of, 59-62
risk factors of, 51-55
victimization experiences, 74
Sexual identity development, 67-85. *See also* Victimization experiences (mental health, revictimization, and sexual identity development issues)
Sexual orientation-religious identity integration, 112
Sexuality feelings, 38-42
Simoni, J. M., 49-66
Social support
buffer effects of, 58
HIV-positive populations, 56-57
socially supportive relationships, 101

Sociodemographics, 58-59
Southern Baptist Convention, 115-118
Spiritual resources, 120
St. Louis County FDVC (Family and Domestic Violence Council), 135-137
St. Louis Lesbian and Gay AVP (Anti-Violence Project), 127-138
Stability (emotional), 99-100
Studies
  of black populations (multiple minority stress and resilience issues), 88-104
  of "coming out" process-related issues, 32-45
  of community interventions (homophobic and partner violence-related issues), 128-134
  of HIV-positive populations (abuse, support, and depression issues), 49-66
  of St. Louis Lesbian and Gay AVP (Anti-Violence Project), 128-134
  of victimization experiences (mental health, revictimization, and sexual identity development issues), 67-85
  of youth populations (developmental challenges and victimization experiences), 9-28
Support-related issues
  HIV-positive populations, 49-66. *See also* HIV-positive populations (abuse, support, and depression issues)
  supportive relationships, 101
Symptoms
  depressive symptomologies, 56
  predictors of, 10, 24

Theoretical frameworks, 89-91
Therapeutic relationships, 119-120
Therapy (conversion), 109,115,118
Transformation and empowerment issues, 118-119
Trauma, stress, and resilience issues. *See also under individual topics*
  black populations (multiple minority stress and resilience issues), 82-108
  "coming out" process-related issues, 31-47
  community interventions (homophobic and partner violence-related issues), 125-139
  HIV-positive populations (abuse, support, and depression issues), 49-66
  institutionalized Judeo-Christian religion issues, 109-123
  introduction to, 1-8
  reference and research resources (general) for, 8
  victimization experiences (mental health, revictimization, and sexual identity development issues), 67-85
  youth populations (developmental challenges and victimization experiences), 9-29
Trustworthiness issues, 93

United Methodist Church, 115-118
U.S. Attorney General (Hate Crimes Task Force), 136

Victimization experiences (mental health, revictimization, and sexual identity development issues)
  CSA (childhood sexual abuse), 77-78
  future perspectives of, 82-83

historical perspectives of, 68-70
introduction to, 67-68
lesbian identity, 77-78
measures for, 71-73
anti-LBG (lesbian-bisexual-gay) victimization, 72,74
BSI (Brief Symptom Inventory), 72-73,76
GSI (Global Severity Index), 72, 76
LBG (lesbian-bisexual-gay) experience aspects, 72-74
Lesbian Wellness Survey, 71-72
mental health, 72-73
National Lesbian Health Care Survey, 81
violence-related experiences, 71-72,74-76
physical abuse, 74
race and ethnicity differences, 78
reference and research resources for, 83-85
revictimization, 76-77
sexual abuse, 74
studies of, 67-85
discussion of, 78-83
introduction to, 67-70
measures for, 71-73
methods for, 71-73
participant data for, 71,73
procedures for, 71
results of, 73-78
Violence
partner and homophobic, 125-139. *See also* Community interventions (homophobic and partner violence-related issues)
prevalence of, 127-128
violence-related experiences, 71-72, 74-76

Youth populations (developmental challenges and victimization experiences)
adjustment indicators for, 21-25
introduction to, 21-22
sexual orientation correlations, 22-25
symptom predictors, 10, 24
challenges of, 25-28
community relationships of, 14,20, 26-27
disclosures and "coming-out" processes of, 26
family member victimization and, 21
future perspectives of, 27-28
introduction to, 9-10
lifetime victimization experiences and, 14-15, 20-21
measures for, 12-16
BSI (Brief Symptom Inventory), 14-15
community relationships, 14
GSI (Global Severity Index), 14-15, 22-24
lifetime victimization experiences, 14-15
parental relationships, 13-14
RSEI (Rosenberg Self-Esteem Inventory), 14-15
sexual orientation development, 12-13
victimization, 14-15
parental relationships of, 13-14, 17-21,26-27
reference and research resources for, 28-29
self-identification ages of, 10-11, 16-17
sexual orientation development of, 12-13,16-17,21
studies of, 9-28
discussion of, 25-28
introduction to, 9-11
limitations of, 27-28
measures for, 12-16
methods for, 11-16
participant data for, 11-12
results of, 16-25
victimization of, 14-15, 20-21